Child-Centred Music Therapy

Viggo Krüger • Kathleen M. Murphy

Child-Centred Music Therapy

Integrating Best Interest of the Child into Theory, Research, and Practice

palgrave
macmillan

Viggo Krüger
Grieg Academy Music Therapy
Research Center
University of Bergen
Bergen, Norway

Kathleen M. Murphy
Department of Music
State University of New York at
New Paltz
New York, USA

The University of Bergen

ISBN 978-3-031-85723-2 ISBN 978-3-031-85724-9 (eBook)
https://doi.org/10.1007/978-3-031-85724-9

This Palgrave Macmillan imprint is published by the registered company Springer Nature Switzerland AG.
The registered company address is: Gewerbestrasse 11, 6330 Cham, Switzerland

Foreword

"It takes a village to raise a child." This is a well-known African proverb, and it is also true in reverse: It takes a child to raise a village. Children are not only recipients of care and guidance. Children teach, challenge, and grow their communities. They are active change-makers (Sen, 2017). In this sensitively nuanced book, Viggo and Kathy invite music therapists to embrace both perspectives, thoughtfully reassessing their thinking and practice to be aligned with the best interests of the children they work with. This is by no means a simple task. Cultural approaches vary, different contexts demand unique responses, and varying degrees of vulnerability necessitate different strategies. A refined degree of cultural humility and sociocultural attunement are non-negotiable. The authors of this book honestly and wisely explore this complexity while still presenting a path for us to walk along, because we can and must respond to the challenge. By "us," this means all of us as different role players because music therapy entails musicking with, thinking with, responding with, and instigating changes with children and those who play a role in their lives.

A focus on exploring "What's wrong with you?" has shifted due to trauma-informed perspectives in the direction of asking instead, "What has happened to you?" We are now seeing this shift again. As Spandler (2024) argued, emphasizing the question "What has happened to you?" places weight on psychosocial assumptions instead of medicalized ones. Medical reasons *and* psychosocial factors may be at play—or neither—but both questions can risk sidelining people's own understandings and solutions. If we ask (instead of or in addition to the other two questions), "What matters to you?" then children's own knowledge and agency can be placed at the centre, and spaces can be created for a wide range of creative possibilities. As we work in alignment with the best interests of the child, we can use this question as an anchor.

This book advocates for an epistemically just approach, a concept articulated by Fricker (2007). Too often still, children are not recognized as "knowers." They are not always seen to be credible communicators (testimonial injustice) and so their perspectives are not sufficiently included in our body of knowledge (hermeneutical injustice). Epistemic injustice can be seen as a problem of recognition (Medina, 2018). People, in this case children, may not be sufficiently seen or heard, or they may be misrecognized and misunderstood. An epistemically just therapist struggling to fully understand a child's experience does not see the child as lacking the ability to clearly explain themselves but realizes that their own understanding and skills need improving so they can better appreciate the child's expressions (Carel & Kidd, 2014). Children's capacities to communicate their experiences develop relationally. Supportive adults around them create conditions for their voices to be heard and for them to grow in their sense of identity as reliable testifiers (Burroughs & Tollefsen, 2016).

Researchers who engage in child-led studies offer us some useful tools for thinking about how to balance centring the child and creating space for their agency, while still offering appropriate adult support (rather than adult management). They also provide insights for thinking about collaborative meaning-making. Music therapy researchers can be particularly effective at this (even when their studies are not fully child-led), emphasizing the importance of paying close attention to multimodal forms of communication (Klyve & Rolvsjord, 2022), stressing the need to respect children's competencies (Krüger & Stige, 2014), and highlighting adult responsibility to ethically protect children while ensuring their voices are heard (Fairchild & McFerran, 2019). These strategies within child-led and child-informed research approaches can inspire our music therapy practice, as we think about children not as the recipients or subjects of therapeutic interventions but as knowledge creators, designers, and co-designers of therapeutic processes.

Working according to and supporting the best interests of the child is inseparable from the best interests of the system the child is a part of. Health and well-being are constructed, experienced, enacted, and situated within social systems, inseparable from political and ethical issues (Blaxter, 2010). The ecology that a child is developing within is also constantly changing, adapting, and being adapted to (Shelton, 2019). We seek to support conditions that enable children to flourish. This necessitates using a relational lens to attend to children's experiences inside and outside the therapy room, as well as engaging in multi-systemic strategies to bring about positive change.

This book is not a landing place. It is a launching point. As we make progress in working towards honouring the best interests of children, we still grapple with some sticky questions that require ongoing attention. For example, how do we work ethically within our scope of practice while attending to urgent needs that present themselves, such as children arriving for music therapy hungry, and the lack of other professionals (social workers, for example) to refer them and their families to when this is necessary? This question is especially relevant in countries like mine where music therapy is a regulated health profession and where so many service users live in extremely under-resourced areas. How do we create therapy spaces that are safe enough in contexts that are far from safe? How do we open access to music therapy training so that more music therapists will be working with children within their own communities rather than predominantly graduating outsider music therapists who are earnestly seeking to relate, empathize, and serve those whose contexts are very different from their own lived experiences?

The best books offer wisdom and ask questions. They give tools for working better today and invite us all to develop even better strategies for tomorrow. This book has lived with me long after I closed the last page. It continues to provoke and inspire me, and I have no doubt that it will do the same for you.

Johannesburg, South Africa — Andeline dos Santos

References

Sen, S. (2017). *Image: No child left invisible.* Harper Collins.

Spandler, H. (2024). "What matters to you?"—An antidote to "What's wrong" and "What happened". *Mad in America: Science, psychiatry and social justice.*

Fricker, M. (2007). *Epistemic injustice. Power and the ethics of knowing.* Oxford University.

Medina, J. (2018). Misrecognition and epistemic injustice. *Feminist Philosophy Quarterly, 4*(4). https://doi.org/10.5206/fpq/2018.4.6233

Burroughs, M. D., & Tollefsen, D. (2016). Learning to listen: Epistemic injustice and the child. *Episteme, 13*(3), 359–377.

Klyve, G. P., & Rolvsjord, R. (2022). Moments of fun: Narratives of children's experiences of music therapy in mental health care. *Nordic Journal of Music Therapy, 32*(2), 100–120. https://doi.org/10.1080/08098131.2022.2055114

Fairchild, R., & McFerran, K. S. (2019). "Music is everything": Using collaborative group songwriting as an arts-based method with children experiencing homelessness and family violence. *Nordic Journal of Music Therapy, 28*(2), 88–107. https://doi.org/10.1080/08098131.2018.1530189

Blaxter, M. (2010). *Health.* Polity.

Shelton, L. (2019). *The Bronfenbrenner primer: A guide to develecology.* Routledge.

Preface

Know your rights.
(The Clash)

This book highlights children's rights to access music therapy when it is in their best interest, using Article 3 of the United Nations Convention on the Rights of the Child (UNCRC, 1989) as a foundational framework. In outlining a child-centered music therapy approach, inspired by Article 3, the principle of the child's best interests, we wish to contribute to an increased awareness of the potential link between human rights for children and music therapy. Article 3 states that all parties, including families, institutions, and public/private agencies, must place the needs of the children they serve at the forefront.

The best interest of the child ensures that children are recognized as "active agents, drawing on their resources and competencies" (Jones et al., 2021). In work with children, gaps may exist between rights and realities, as noted by Krüger and Stige (2014), highlighting the importance of raising awareness of children's rights in music therapy research, theory, and practice.

> The situation of adolescents under welfare care is in many ways at odds with the rights and values of the Convention on the Rights of the Child (…) the values of the UNCRC are highly relevant in relation to music therapy and child welfare, but these values are often neglected in music therapy research, theory and practice. (p. 2)

In terms of music therapy, music can be a way for children to promote their identity and hence their own life story, for better or worse. Song lyrics, affiliations with genres or artists, and the use of social media are technologies in the formation, articulation, and performance of the child's own voice. As such, the many songs, performances, and improvisations created within music therapy sessions can highlight children's rights and offer platforms for performances that showcase the best interest of the child.

The best interest of the child is dependent upon how the concept is understood and realized in each culture or setting. Different cultural approaches will inevitably outline different understandings of what is in a child's best interests. This means that what is in the best interest of a child can vary depending on the sociocultural circumstances, cultural norms, societal values, and the specific needs of the child. Hence, the principle recognizes that there is no one-size-fits-all approach and requires an assessment appropriate to the specific context of the child. Decisions should be made by considering the unique context of each child's situation as definitions of health, cultural diversity, economic conditions, and socioeconomic factors influence what is "best" for a child's well-being. The book is built on a value framework promoting the view that when assessing the child's best interests regarding music therapy experiences, planning, implementation, and assessment should be conducted on a case-by-case basis, considering the specific circumstances of each child or group of children. Determining what is in the best interest of the child often involves navigating conflicting interests, such as those between the child's interests and those of adults or between individual care and societal interests.

Since the end of World War II, music therapy has significantly evolved as a recognized profession, practice, and academic discipline across many countries (Ruud, 1998). The growth of academic programmes has fostered a rich scholarly environment (Goodman, 2011), and the practice of music therapy has expanded over the years, with approximately 12,000 music therapists currently working with diverse populations worldwide. Among these professionals, about one-third specialize in working with children and adolescents under the age of 18, indicating a substantial commitment to addressing the unique needs of this population (Kern & Tague, 2017).

The involvement of music therapists in the lives of children and adolescents extends beyond individual therapy sessions. Music therapists often work in collaboration with other professionals, such as educators, social workers, psychologists, and healthcare providers, to create co-support systems for young individuals. This interdisciplinary approach enhances the overall effectiveness of therapeutic interventions, as it allows for a more holistic understanding of each child's or adolescent's needs (McFerran, 2020). Furthermore, the impact of music therapy is not limited to the therapist and the client alone. Family members and friends play a crucial role in the therapeutic process, as their involvement can significantly influence the outcomes of therapy. Engaging parents and guardians in music therapy sessions fosters a supportive environment where children and adolescents can express themselves more freely. Involvement like this helps caregivers understand the therapeutic processes and strategies that can be applied at home, reinforcing the skills learned during sessions. In addition to direct interactions with clients, music therapists often participate in community outreach and educational programmes aimed at raising awareness about the benefits of music therapy. These initiatives can involve workshops, presentations, and group activities designed to demonstrate the therapeutic potential of music in various contexts. By reaching out to broader audiences, music therapists can cultivate a deeper understanding of the field and encourage more individuals to explore its benefits.

However, the link between the UNCRC and music therapy is yet to be fully formulated in a book unlike what has been published in other professions (e.g. Gillett-Swan et al., 2021; Urban et al., 2022). For this reason, we ask the following questions: (1) *How does Article 3 of the United Nations Convention on the Rights of the Child (UNCRC), which emphasizes the best interests of the child, relate to the practice and application of music therapy?*, and (2) *what are the implications for research and practice?* We have chosen to focus on Article 3 of the UNCRC as this article relates to all the other articles. It has been argued that Article 3 underpins all the other provisions of the Convention (Ruggiero, 2022).

> The best interests are one of the most complicated concepts to pin down, and the Committee defines it as 'a dynamic concept that requires an assessment appropriate to the specific context.' What is encompassed by best interests depends on how the concept is understood. (p. 23)

In the book we take part in an international discourse known as a best interest of the child perspective (Falch-Eriksen & Backe Hansen, 2018). A best interest of the child perspective takes as a point of departure for understanding children's rights and the interests of various stakeholders, such as adults, institutions, or even society. This perspective allows viewing children's rights in relation to broader societal interests and priorities. Rights can be weighed against other considerations, such as economic interests or political objectives. Using this perspective might prioritize the interests of adults over the genuine needs and rights of children. A need perspective, on the other hand, prioritizes the inherent needs and rights of children themselves as the primary focus of attention. It emphasizes recognizing and fulfilling the fundamental needs of children, such as the right to education, healthcare, protection from violence and exploitation, and opportunities for development and participation. Advocates of the need perspective argue for a child-centred approach to policymaking and decision-making, where the best interests of the child are paramount and guides all actions and interventions. Throughout the book, we balance the discussion closely related to how we perceive the child within a sociocultural context, advocating for both an interest and a need perspective.

Assessment for determining the best interest of the child involves weighing the above-mentioned elements to find the best approach (GC No. 14, CRC, 2013). Jensen et al. (2022) offer suggestions on how to promote a child-friendly approach in working with children based on the best interest of the child approach. Their report from the PARTICIPATION project focuses on mapping and evaluating existing child protection structures while identifying factors that both hinder and facilitate children's involvement. They recommend clear, balanced guidelines to help professionals promote and assess inclusive participation, considering children's ability, gender identity, sexual orientation, and socioeconomic background. The guidelines should enhance awareness of information provision and discourage assumptions about children's knowledge. Professionals are urged to clarify how they weigh and document children's opinions in decision-making and foster diverse communication methods, beyond verbal exchanges, for more meaningful engagement. Building trust with children requires time and resources, and reducing adult–child power imbalances is essential to ensuring children's voices are genuinely valued in decisions.[1].

[1] As an attempt to meet the criteria outlined in the report, we have developed a guideline for the use of music therapy with children, which is attached as an appendix on page 179. This guideline is the result of a thorough review of available research on music therapy, relevant theories, and the principles of the UNCRC.

Research on participation and assessment in music therapy, as well as related professions, remains limited (Johansen & Bonde, 2020). The existing literature on assessments for use in music therapy settings is outdated. For example, Aitchison and Skewes McFerran (2023) highlighted a significant gap in assessment tools tailored specifically for adolescent mental health. Moreover, they observed that many of the existing publications were produced before the widespread adoption of human rights-, participatory-oriented care models and do not reflect a best interest of the child framework. This misalignment underscores the need for updated tools and approaches that prioritize children's rights and well-being within therapeutic assessments, particularly in adolescent mental health contexts.

Who Is This Book For?

This book serves as a comprehensive guide for those dedicated to improving the lives of children and adolescents through the transformative power of music, fostering interdisciplinary collaboration and innovative practices across various fields. This book is relevant for anyone interested in the intersection of human rights, music, and children, particularly those who work with or involve children and adolescents in their research including music therapists, teachers, social workers, nurses, lawyers, and others. For example, the book provides critical insights that are relevant for music therapists, as it elucidates the therapeutic potential of music in promoting children's rights and enhancing their overall well-being. It can be a resource for individuals engaged in the intersection of human rights, music, and childhood studies. Educators may find the text beneficial in identifying strategies to incorporate music into pedagogical practices that foster inclusive and supportive learning environments. Social workers can leverage the book's content to understand how music can serve as a mechanism for advocacy and empowerment, particularly when working with marginalized populations. Similarly, healthcare professionals, including nurses and doctors, can gain insights into the role of music in enhancing patient care and providing emotional support to children facing health challenges. Lastly, legal practitioners specializing in child advocacy will find discussions within the book pertinent to navigating the legal frameworks that uphold children's rights through artistic expression.

The Aim of the Book and Literature Review Strategy

The aim of this book is to review research published during the twenty-first century in which children were research participants. We explore how current research contributes to the discourse on the best interest of the child. The literature review was conducted by searching for themes related to music therapy and the best interests of the child in five databases: RILM Abstracts of Music Literature (Ebsco), ERIC (Ebsco), MEDLINE (Ovid), APA PsycInfo (Ovid), and Web of Science (Clarivate). Search terms included free text term or subject headings for "music therapy", combined with child-related terms (e.g. child*, "young people," adolescence) and thematic search terms relevant to child welfare and rights (e.g. "best interest of the child," "children's voice," "participation"). Each search focused on materials published between 2007 and 2024, with a particular emphasis on recent literature in English.

Music therapy practice often addresses issues related to children's health, well-being, education, and democratic participation. In reviewing the research and writings related to music therapy practice with children we highlight paradoxes and ambivalences that music therapy practitioners and researchers encounter when striving to determine what is in the best interests of the child. We believe that when planning any activity involving music and music therapy, the United Nations Convention on the Rights of the Child (UNCRC), particularly the best interest of the child, is a natural (and just) starting point (United Nations, 1989). General human rights ensure that every human being, including children, is allowed civil and political rights to live in an open and free society (Kilkelly & Liefaard, 2019). However, why do we have specific human rights for children? One answer lies in children's potentially fragile status as human beings and their need for age-appropriate solutions. Children's rights are human rights adapted specifically to children because societies must consider the child's developmental needs over time.

In sum, we hope the research and clinical work described in this book will demonstrate how music therapists can uphold the spirit of the UNCRC while working within the constraints of their clinical settings. Additionally, we hope that readers are inspired to advocate for change so that all children who would benefit have access to music therapy.

Overview of the Book

This book explores the intersection of music therapy with the best interest of the child, grounded in various theoretical frameworks, interdisciplinary insights, and real-world practices. It aims to provide an extensive understanding of how music therapy can serve children's rights and well-being across diverse contexts, from family care to educational and mental health settings. The chapters are designed to guide music therapists, educators, and interdisciplinary teams through the intricacies of child welfare and protection through a music therapy lens.

Part I outlines a rights-based theoretical framework based on sociocultural perspectives and critical childhood studies. The section will review some historical events describing why the best interest of the child is a prominent guiding framework. Following a sociocultural theory framework, we understand the best interest of the child as interwoven with many layers and levels, involving a wide variety of implications for practice and research. Chapter 1 sets the historical and geographical context, discussing how children's rights and the role of music align with the best interest of the child. This chapter provides a historical overview of The UN Convention on the Rights of the Child (UNCRC), concentrating more specifically on Article 3 (United Nations, 1989). We highlight an increasing interest in the field of music therapy and children's rights during the last two decades. The chapter also addresses critiques of the concept and sets up the foundation for further exploration. Chapter 2 describes key factors that influence a child's best interest, such as the child's identity, cultural sensitivity, family preservation, and protection in vulnerable situations. The chapter explains the role of professional judgement in assessing and determining best interest of child practices in music therapy. We are especially interested in how music therapy facilitates a holistic and contextualized view on how the best interest of the child can be assessed and determined through processes of professional judgement. Chapter 2 also examines the role of music therapy within Best Interest Determination (BID) processes. BID addresses individual needs, stakeholder collaboration, systemic influences, and the societal factors that impact child welfare, while considering challenges like cultural competence and communication barriers. Chapter 3 introduces sociocultural perspectives, discussing resource-oriented, culture-centred, and community music therapy. Trauma and resilience-informed approaches, critical childhood studies, and the role of music therapy in social justice are highlighted. Moreover, the chapter explores sociocultural perspectives and inspirations from critical childhood studies. We argue that music therapy is best understood by considering multidisciplinary approaches, incorporating critical thinking in line with perspectives from post-humanism.

In Part II, we draw on music therapy research from various populations. The aim of this section is not to cover all research conducted regarding children, but rather to highlight research that we find relevant in terms of the best interest of the child. The main goal of this chapter is to identify key aspects of music therapy practices that align with the best interest of the child. Chapter 4 explores the role of music therapy in family care, including alternative care models like foster care, adoption, and residential care. Gaps in research and recommendations for practice are identified. Chapter 5[2] covers the integration of music therapy into educational and broader cultural frameworks, enhancing the development and well-being of children in school environments. Chapter 6 addresses the role of music therapy in both inpatient and outpatient mental health care. It includes discussions on sensitive topics such as freedom from sexual abuse, minor migrants, and music therapy for sex offenders, identifying areas where further research is needed. Chapter 7 focuses on paediatric care, reviewing music therapy interventions designed for children and adolescents, and their families, in medical settings. Part III outlines implications for research as well as providing a summary of the book's main ideas. Chapter 8 provides guidance for ethical research that meets criteria set forth in the UNCRC and follows a "best interest of the child" philosophy. Chapter 9 ties together practical and theoretical insights, encouraging the integration of music therapy practices with established frameworks and policies aimed at safeguarding the best interests of the child.

Bergen, Norway — Viggo Krüger
New York, NY, USA — Kathleen M. Murphy

References

Carel, H., & Kidd, I. J. (2014). Epistemic injustice in healthcare: A philosophial analysis. *Medicine, Health Care and Philosophy, 17*, 529–540.

Falch-Eriksen, A., & Backe-Hansen, E. (2018). Child protection and human rights: A call for professional practice and policy. In A. Falch-Eriksen &

[2] Chapter 5 is written by Maren Metell.

E. Backe-Hansen (Eds.), *Human rights in child protection: Implications for professional practice* (pp. 1–15). Palgrave Macmillan.

Gillett-Swan, J., Thelander, N., & Hanna, A. (2021). Setting the scene for children's rights and education: Understanding the aims of education. In J. Gillett-Swan & N. Thelander (Eds.), *Children's rights from international educational perspectives* (Transdisciplinary Perspectives in Educational Research) (Vol. 2). Springer. https://doi.org/10.1007/978-3-030-80861-7_1

Goodman, K. D. (2011). *Music therapy education and training: From theory to practice*. Charles C. Thomas Publisher.

Jensen, F. P., Križ, K., & Skivenes, M. (2022, July 11). *Structuring practice for children's participation: Report I for the participation project: Mapping and evaluating organizational guidelines*. Centre for Research on Discretion and Paternalism, University of Bergen.

Johansson, K., & Bonde, L. O. (Ed.). (2000). *Music in Paediatric Hospitals: Nordic Perspectives*. CREMAH.

Jones, P., Cedar, L., Coleman, A., Haythorne, D., Mercieca, D., & Ramsden, E. (2021). *Child agency and voice in therapy: New ways of working in the arts therapies*. Routledge.

Kern, P., & Tague, D. (2017). Music therapy practice status and trends worldwide: An international survey study. *Music Therapy Perspectives, 35*(1), 255–286. https://doi.org/10.1093/jmt/thx011

Kilkelly, U., & Liefaard, T. (2019). International human rights of children. In *International human rights* (pp. 138–154). Springer.

Krüger, V., & Stige, B. (2014). Between rights and realities—Music as a structuring resource in the context of child welfare aftercare. A qualitative study. *Nordic Journal of Music Therapy, 24*(2), 1–24.

McFerran, K. S. (2020). Adolescents and music therapy: Contextualized recommendations for research and practice. *Music Therapy Perspectives, 38*(1), 80–88. https://doi.org/10.1093/mtp/miz014

Ruggiero, R. (2022). Article 3: The Best Interest of the Child, In Vaghri, Z. (2022). Monitoring state compliance with the UN Convention on the rights of the child. *Children's Well-Being: Indicators and Research, 25*. https://doi.org/10.1007/978-3-030-84647-3_3

Ruud, E. (1998). *Music therapy, improvisation, communication, and culture*. Barcelona Publishers.

UN Committee on the Rights of the Child (UNCRC). (2013). *General comment No. 14 on the right of the child to have his or her best interests taken as a primary consideration (art. 3, para. 1)*. CRC/C/GC/14. Retrieved from https://www2.ohchr.org/english/bodies/crc/docs/gc/crc_c_gc_14_eng.pdf

United Nations. (1989). *Convention on the rights of the child*. https://www.ohchr.org/en/instruments-mechanisms/instruments/convention-rights-child

United Nations (UNCRC) (1989). *Convention on the rights of the child*. https://www.ohchr.org/en/instrumentsmechanisms/instruments/convetion-rights-child

Urban, M., Fairchild, N., Vandenbroeck, M., Lenz Taguchi, H., & Macrine, S. (Eds.). (2022). *Reconceptualising children's rights in infant-toddler care and education: Transnational conversations*. Springer. https://doi.org/10.1007/978-3-031-05218-7

Acknowledgements

We would like to express our heartfelt gratitude to everyone who has supported us throughout this journey. First and foremost, we extend our sincere thanks to the twin centres—GAMUT, or the Grieg Academy Music Therapy Research Centre at the University of Bergen, and the Norwegian research centre NORCE—for providing an inspiring environment that fosters innovative research and collaboration. Your commitment to advancing the field of music therapy for children and adolescents has been invaluable.

We also wish to acknowledge the Centre for Discretion and Paternalism at the University of Bergen for their resources, which have greatly enriched this work. Their expertise has deepened our understanding of the complexities within our field.

To our colleagues and family, your support, encouragement, and constructive feedback have been instrumental in shaping this project.

Finally, this book has been published with financial support from the Faculty of Fine Art, Music, and Design at the University of Bergen, as well as the Publication Fund for Open Access at the University of Bergen.

Thanks to academic librarian Regina Küfner Lein at the Medical library, University in Bergen for discussing search terms, running the searches, and deduplication of records.

Contents

About the Authors

Viggo Krüger has over 25 years of experience in the field of music therapy, serving as both a research leader and professor at the Grieg Academy Music Therapy Research Centre at the University of Bergen, as well as at NORCE (Norwegian Research Centre). His dual roles in academia and research position him as a key contributor to the advancement of music therapy practices and knowledge, particularly in Norway. Krüger's scholarly contributions encompass numerous books, book chapters, and articles. He is a past chair of the Norwegian Music Therapy Association and has held several roles and positions in the development of music therapy in Norway.

Kathleen M. Murphy is an associate professor and Programme Director, Music Therapy Graduate Studies at the State University of New York at New Paltz. She is a licensed creative arts therapist (LCAT) and Board-Certified Music Therapist (MT-BC). She has over 40 years of clinical and research experience. She has written and presented nationally and internationally on a variety of topics related to music therapy clinical practice, education, and supervision. Her research interests are focused on music therapy in substance dependence across the lifespan, trauma, and community music therapy. She is a member of the Association for Music and Imagery, the non-profit organization Public Responsibility in Medicine & Research, the International Association for Music and Medicine and the American Music Therapy Association, where she has served in leadership positions on the state, regional, and national levels. Currently, she serves as member of AMTA's Academic Program Approval Committee.

Maren Metell is a postdoctoral fellow in music therapy at the Grieg Academy, Faculty for Fine Arts, Music and Design, University of Bergen. She has worked with children and families in pedagogical and community settings. Her research interests include dimensions of power in music therapy, children's access to music, and participatory and arts-based approaches.

PART I

The Best Interest of the Child and Its Relevance for Music Therapy

CHAPTER 1

Situating the Best Interest of the Child and Its Relevance for Music Therapy

Introduction

"In all actions"

"In all actions" includes decisions, acts, conducts, proposals, services, procedures, and other measures including inaction and omissions.

"Concerning"

"Concerning" refers to the forms of actions that directly and indirectly affect children. Furthermore, "concerning" must be interpreted inclusively as relevant to, with an impact on children or affecting children.

"Shall be"

The term "shall be" implies that the states parties have strong legal obligations.

(*continued*)

V. Krüger, K. M. Murphy, *Child-Centred Music Therapy*,
https://doi.org/10.1007/978-3-031-85724-9_1

(continued)

"A primary consideration"

"The best interests of the child" principle shall be "a primary consideration," which provides for special protection of children in any context and acknowledges their unique vulnerability. The principle is of non-derogable nature, which means it does not allow for limitations even in times of emergencies (Committee on the Rights of the Child, 2013).

In writing this book, we are proposing a specific view on how we believe children should be approached in music therapy. Consequently, our perspective is not neutral but value laden. Our values are grounded in the United Nations Convention on the Rights of the Child (UNCRC, 1989), particularly Article 3, which emphasizes the best interests of the child (United Nations, 1989). By adopting this perspective, we position ourselves within a particular discourse—the human rights discourse for children.

The best interest of the child is a core principle in all matters concerning children, whether at the individual, institutional, or societal level. This principle applies to a wide range of contexts, including family life, schools, welfare systems, and healthcare, as well as practices and research involving children (Falch-Eriksen & Backe-Hansen, 2018). Central to this principle is the recognition of children as active agents with the right to influence policies that affect them, helping to shape a just and democratic society grounded in human rights values (Skivenes & Sørsdal, 2018). More broadly, a right can be understood as a legal or moral entitlement granted by a constitution, statute, regulation, judicial precedent, or other legal frameworks. With these rights come corresponding duties and responsibilities, which are integral to upholding justice and equity in society.

The UNCRC does not offer a precise definition of what the best interest of the child is (United Nations, 1989). While the term "best interests" broadly describes the well-being of a child, it is not possible to give a conclusive definition of what is in the best interests of the child, as this depends on a variety of individual circumstances, such as the age and the level of maturity of the child, the presence or absence of parents, and the child's environment. The UNCRC applies to all children in general, in all countries and cultures, and all children around the globe have a right to childhood, not solely those with available resources. The Committee on the Rights of the Child (UNICEF, GC No. 14, 2013) recommends that (1) the content of the UNCRC should be translated into relevant languages, (2) child-friendly/appropriate versions should be made available, (3) conferences, seminars, workshops, and other events should be held to disseminate guidelines for implementation, and (4) it be incorporated into the formal pre- and in-service training of all concerned professionals and technical staff.

UNCRC Definition of How Long a Child Should Be Protected

The UNCRC protects the rights of children and young people under the age of 18 (United Nations, 1989). However, in some countries, like Norway, the age limit for specific protections is extended up to 25, particularly for vulnerable young adults requiring assistance during their transition to independence. For example, Norway's *Child Welfare Act* allows continued support for young people in care beyond 18 (Barnevernloven, Section 1–3). Other countries have similar provisions. In the UK, the *Children and Families Act 2014* extends care support until 25 (Children and Families Act, 2014). In Canada, Ontario's *Children, Youth and Family Services Act* (2017) and British Columbia's *Agreements with Young Adults* (AYAs) programme also provide extended support until 24–25 (Children, Youth and Family Services Act, 2017; British Columbia Ministry of Children and Family Development). Australia's *Home Stretch* programme supports young people until 21 in states like Victoria (Victorian Government, 2018), and New Zealand amended the *Oranga Tamariki Act* 1989 to extend care up to 25 (Oranga Tamariki, 1989/2019). These policies reflect the growing recognition that many young people require extended care beyond 18 to achieve full independence. In line with this, music therapy service provision should extend beyond the age of 18 to ensure that the therapeutic benefits continue to support the best interests of young adults as they transition into adulthood.

Historical and Geographical Background

The concept of children's rights as we know it today has long historical roots. Looking back in time, Aristotle believed that childhood was a crucial period in human development, during which a person's physical, mental, and emotional faculties were shaped. In his work "Politics," Aristotle outlined his views on the education of children. He believed that education should be tailored to the individual needs of each child, considering their natural abilities, interests, and strengths (Aristotle, 2015). Recent studies in archaeology show an increasing interest in historical perspectives on children and conditions for child rearing (Eriksen, 2017). From a medieval Scandinavian context, the Vikings viewed children as a blessing and a source of great joy to their families. They believed that children were gifts from the Gods, and they were proud of their children's accomplishments. Children were given much love and affection and were taught how to live a life of honour and courage. Children were encouraged to participate in sports and activities. They were also taught the importance of hard work and loyalty. The Viking King Olav is often regarded as a children's rights protector, and in an old law text we find the following statement:

> that every child that is born in our land shall be reared [and cared for], O[laf] : unless it be born with some serious deformity, the face turned around to where the neck should be, or the toes to where the heel should be; in such a case the child shall be brought to church to be baptized, and then [it may be] laid down in the church and be left to perish. (Simensen, 2021, p. 45, Chapter 21)

Even though we can find interesting traces of children's rights in ancient readings, the timeline for the modern history of children's rights can be traced back to around 1600, and the Elizabethan "Poor Law." The Elizabethan Poor Law of 1601 established a system to aid the poor in England and Wales, providing indoor relief in workhouses and outdoor relief through money, food, or clothing. It aimed to support those unable to work, like the elderly and children (Hindle, 2000). The first international agreement on children's rights, the Declaration of the Rights of the Child, was signed in Geneva, Switzerland, in 1841. In 1893, the Massachusetts Supreme Court recognized the concept of "the best interests of the child" in child custody cases. In 1924, an amendment to the US Constitution known as the "Child Labor Amendment" was introduced. This amendment called for a ban on the employment of children under the age of 14.

The concept of "best interest of the child" was introduced by Eglantyne Jebb (1876–1928) who founded Save the Children in 1919 (Jebb, 1924). The phenomenon of the "angel maker" offers a dark historical context to reflect on the evolution of child rights explaining the harsh realities of the time. Angel makers were individuals, often women, who engaged in infanticide or child neglect, typically within the practice of baby farming (Jones, 2002; Kilday & Nash, 2023). This practice emerged out of dire poverty, lack of social welfare, and the absence of legal protection for children during the nineteenth century, when unwanted infants—often from poor, single mothers—were handed over to these caregivers in exchange for money. Many of these children perished due to malnutrition, neglect, or outright murder, highlighting the complete absence of safeguards for children's well-being.

Jebb's work arose in response to the devastating conditions children faced during and after World War I. Children were among the most vulnerable victims of conflict, famine, and neglect, paralleling the earlier plight of children during Victorian times, when practices like baby farming and angel making exposed the severe lack of protection and care for vulnerable young lives. Jebb wrote the "Declaration of the Rights of the Child," which served as a precursor to the United Nations Convention on the Rights of the Child (Jebb, 1924).

- The child must be given the means requisite for its normal development, both materially and spiritually.
- The child that is hungry must be fed, the child that is sick must be nursed, the child that is backward must be helped, the delinquent child must be reclaimed, and the orphan and the waif must be sheltered and succoured.
- The child must be the first to receive relief in times of distress.
- The child must be put in a position to earn a livelihood and must be protected against every form of exploitation.
- The child must be brought up in the consciousness that its talents must be devoted to the service of its fellow men. (p. 1)

The Declaration of the Rights of the Child emphasized the importance of children's well-being, protection, and development, and it called for special safeguards and care for children in need. Jebb's advocacy work helped raise awareness about the plight of children during and after times of conflict and paved the way for the modern understanding of children's rights. Finally, in 1959, the best interest of the child was formalized in the United Nations (UN) Declaration of the Rights of the Child (para. 2) (United Nations General Assembly, 1959). The Declaration of the Rights of the Child emphasized the need for special care and protection for children, including appropriate legal protection before and after birth, outlined in the document as ten principles:

- **Equality**: The right to equality, without distinction on account of race, religion, or national origin.
- **Special Protection**: The right to special protection for the child's physical, mental, and social development.
- **Identity**: The right to a name and a nationality.
- **Basic Needs**: The right to adequate nutrition, housing, and medical services.
- **Special Education and Treatment**: The right to special education and treatment when a child is physically or mentally handicapped.
- **Love and Understanding**: The right to understanding and love by parents and society.
- **Recreation and Education**: The right to recreational activities and free education.
- **Priority in Relief**: The right to be among the first to receive relief in all circumstances.
- **Protection from Harm**: The right to protection against all forms of neglect, cruelty, and exploitation.
- **Spirit of Brotherhood**: The right to be brought up in a spirit of understanding, tolerance, friendship among peoples, and universal brotherhood (p. 1).

The declaration from 1959 led to the creation and adoption of the 1989 UN Convention on the Rights of the Child (United Nations, 1989). This document outlines the rights of all children worldwide. The UNCRC are formulated as individual, universal, and moral rights. Like human rights, the convention is based on values such as autonomy, equality, and equality. The UNCRC can be regarded as a tool meant to provide guidance for all children and their families. According to the UNCRC, children, as rights holders, are entitled not only to protection, provision, and participation as established by the UN Convention on the Rights of the Child (UNCRC), but they also bear a responsibility to respect and uphold the rights of others. This view promotes the idea that children, through their actions, can actively contribute to the realization of their peers' rights, demonstrating empathy and responsibility in everyday interactions. Whether standing against bullying, advocating for inclusivity, or supporting marginalized peers, children can engage meaningfully in fostering a rights-respecting community. This concept of children's responsibility is essential in nurturing future citizens who are socially aware and committed to safeguarding the rights of all (Lansdown, 2011).

The convention is relevant for professions in health, educational and social work, including music therapy. The UNCRC affects all children in general, in all countries and culture. It implies a holistic, universal, and value-based view of childhood. Instead of solely looking at childhood as a biological, natural state, childhood is understood to be culturally constructed. Responsibility that the best interest of the child is taken care of is placed on all adults, not just professionals (United Nations, 1989). All children around the globe have a right to childhood, not solely those with available resources.

Music Therapy and Children's Rights

From a socio-historical perspective, human practices such as holding, dancing, singing, creating images, storytelling, and sharing celebrations and family rituals have long been recognized as promoting healthy well-being and healing (Small, 1998), but the interest in the connection between children's rights and music is a rather new one (Stige & Aarø, 2012). One point of departure could be to argue that the interest for the link between children's rights and music therapy started in 2012. "The

Children's Right to Music project," a pioneering work by Curtis and Vaillancourt (2012), was designed as a multifaceted programme to increase awareness of human rights and to promote resource and skill development in ensuring these rights are upheld, specifically about the rights of children with disabilities. As the authors describe, the programme was designed to meet the following objectives:

- To increase awareness of the rights of children with disabilities as outlined in the Convention on the Rights of Children and in the Convention on the Rights of People with Disabilities.
- To increase an understanding of the implication of these rights as they pertain to children with disabilities' right to music, music-making, and active participation in the community, within the full scope of its social and cultural life; and
- To increase understanding of, resources for, and skills in making music accessible to children with disabilities (Curtis & Vaillancourt, 2012, p. 7).

Across various countries, music therapy researchers have aligned their work with the principles of the UNCRC. One notable example is Finnish music therapist Hakomäki (2012), who connects music therapy to Article 12 of the convention, which emphasizes the right of children to express their views freely in matters affecting them. Hakomäki describes how participation in music therapy, particularly through songwriting and performance, provides children with space for self-expression, enabling them to share their thoughts and emotions in a creative, non-verbal manner. Using music therapy in this way becomes especially powerful when working with children who may find it difficult to articulate their feelings through traditional methods.

Another example comes from Norwegian psychologist Helle-Valle (2016), who provides music activities within a kindergarten setting. Her research also draws on the UNCRC, focusing on how music activities can empower children to express themselves and challenge societal labels. Specifically, Helle-Valle discusses the use of music activities to help children diagnosed with ADHD create an alternative identity. Through musical activities, these children can present themselves beyond the limitations of the ADHD diagnosis, forming what Helle-Valle refers to as an "AD/HD Identity" in their community. This approach aligns with the UNCRC's focus on children's right to be active participants in their own lives and communities. In her opinion there is a tension between the UNCRC and the ADHD diagnoses given to many children, she states:

> the tension between being seen and heard oneself vs. being aware of others and of community can be understood considering tension between the Convention on the Rights of the Child (United Nations, 1989), where children's rights to be seen and heard are described, and the descriptions of how children's should not behave (e.g., the ADHD diagnosis). (p. 9)

Enge and Stige (2022) highlight the crucial role schools play in protecting and advancing the rights of refugee children. They argue that schools are key spaces for providing not only education but also emotional and psychological support. By incorporating music therapy and creative arts into the curriculum, schools can help refugee children adjust, express themselves, and integrate socially. Their work calls for a focus on the mental health and well-being of refugee children, ensuring their right to education is met in a comprehensive and inclusive way. They reference Article 29 of the UNCRC (1989), which asserts that:

> ...the education of the child shall be directed to the development of the child's personality, talents and mental and physical abilities to their fullest potential. (p. 3)

Klyve and Rolvsjord (2022) emphasize the importance of creating environments where children are viewed as capable of forming and expressing their own views, regardless of their age. They argue that children should be recognized as individuals with their own perspectives and seen as active participants in their lives, which requires a genuine commitment to understanding children's communication. Metell (2023) explores the right to music for children with disabilities, highlighting how music can create accessible spaces for self-expression and participation. Her work stresses the importance of ensuring that all children, regardless of ability, can engage with music in a meaningful way. Fairchild and Mraz (2018) discuss the significance of the UNCRC, particularly the right to be heard, in relation to children who have experienced family violence. They highlight the importance of upholding these children's rights to express their views and to be seen as active agents in their own lives. Similarly, Fairchild et al. (2017) conducted an interpretative synthesis of the literature to examine how children experiencing homelessness are described. Their work emphasizes the importance of recognizing these children as individuals with agency rather than as passive victims. This aligns with the principles of the UNCRC (1989), as their project seeks to affirm children's right to be heard and to freely voice their perspectives on issues that directly affect their lives. From a Brazilian context, Oselame (2023) explore the use of music therapy with adolescents in a detention centre in Brazil, aligning her research with the principles of the UNCRC (1989). Female adolescents aged 15–18 years, who used music therapy not only as a means of emotional expression but also as a tool to strengthen their social connections participated in this study. Through active participation in songwriting, performance, and collaborative music-making, the girls were able to amplify their voices, sharing their experiences and perspectives. Oselame's study highlights how participation in music therapy can raise awareness of children's rights by offering marginalized youth a platform to be heard. This has the potential to empower and foster a sense of belonging and agency, which is essential for rehabilitation and personal growth. This approach underscores the importance of recognizing young people's rights to participation and self-expression, as outlined in the UNCRC (1989), particularly in challenging and restrictive environments like detention centres.

Mitchell (2023), a Canadian music therapist, frames her work within the context of the right to cultural participation, as outlined in the UNCRC. She emphasizes that, in many societies, artistic and cultural experiences are often undervalued, despite the recognition that access to these experiences is a fundamental human right. In her view, music education and music therapy play a crucial role in ensuring that individuals, particularly children, have opportunities to engage with and benefit from artistic activities. Mitchell argues that cultural participation is not merely an enriching experience but a right that fosters creativity, self-expression, and social inclusion. By advocating for the inclusion of music and other artistic forms in educational and therapeutic settings, she highlights the responsibility of music therapists and educators to uphold this right, ensuring that children from all backgrounds have equal access to cultural experiences. Her work underscores the importance of cultural participation in fostering a sense of identity and belonging, particularly in communities where access to the arts may be limited or undervalued.

> In a society that undervalues artistic experience, and yet also recognizes access to such experience as a human right (United Nations Convention on the Rights of the Child, 1989), our work as music educators and music therapists is invaluable. (Mitchell, 2023, p. 45)

The Role of Music Relevant for the Best Interest of the Child

We regard a holistic, contextual approach to music therapy as foundational to the contents of this book. As a medium music is a powerful tool for expression and communication. As such, music is more than just a collection of sounds; it is a powerful sociocultural phenomenon with deep roots in human history (Blacking, 1978). Small (1998) considers "music" to be a verb, not a noun. He understands music as action, not as an object or a thing. Hence, he employs the term "musicking" to propose a paradigm of musical meanings rooted in contextual elements of relationships and ritual. "To music," according to Small (1998), means "to take part, in any capacity, in a musical performance, whether by performing, by listening, by rehearsing or practicing, by providing material for performance (what is called composing), or by dancing" (p. 9). Musicking, according to Small, is a communal and functional human activity that affords people a means to explore, affirm, and celebrate their identities. As such, music carries the ability to adapt, grow, and connect in new ways, continuously reshaping the listener's and performer's experiences. In this way, music reflects the fluidity of life itself (Trehub et al., 2015).

Small's (1998) perspective suggests the true challenge isn't simply about creating more skilled musicians but about fostering environments where informal and formal musical interactions can flourish and contribute to the broader social development and "musicalizing" of society. This resonates with the idea that music has a place not only in traditional venues like concert halls or festivals, but also in everyday settings such as child protection institutions, families, schools, and hospitals. In the context of our book, this view reflects a broad and inclusive approach to music, suggesting that *musicking*—the act of participating in any form of musical activity—can be a valuable tool for enhancing human connection, emotional expression, and community-building in diverse environments. Music becomes a resource for social and personal development, creating spaces for healing, bonding, and empowerment, particularly in contexts of vulnerability or care. This challenges the conventional notion of where and how music belongs, advocating for its integration into all aspects of life and society.

This view is supported by Fancourt and Finn (2019) who believe music can become a resource for health and well-being as well as social participation and learning. The World Health Organization (Fancourt & Finn, 2019) noted that the arts have the potential to impact both mental and physical health across the lifespan, which includes the lives of children. Their findings should be of interest to researchers, policymakers, and practitioners in fields concerning children such as education, child welfare, health, and social work.

Music Therapy Settings and Activities

Music therapy is provided in a variety of settings. Individual music therapy focuses on addressing personal issues, emotional challenges, and mental health concerns in one-on-one sessions between a music therapist and a client. These sessions are tailored to address the specific needs and goals of the individual, whether they be physical, emotional, cognitive, social, or spiritual. Music therapy conducted on an individual level can provide a safe space for individuals to explore their thoughts and feelings, gain insight into their behaviours, and develop coping strategies.

Music therapists use various methods including improvisations, listening, performing, and songwriting to support children's emotional, social, and personal development. For example, improvisation allows children to create music, enabling real-time expression of emotions and thoughts, fostering emotional expression, communication, and creativity. Listening involves engaging children with selected music to encourage reflection on their feelings and experiences, promoting emotional awareness and serving as a conversation starter. Songwriting, either by composing original songs or by adapting existing ones, helps children address specific themes or emotions, encouraging self-expression, storytelling, and emotional processing. Movement to music includes incorporating physical movement in response to music, whether structured or free form, enhancing body awareness, self-regulation, and emotional release. Song discussion involves a holistic exploration of the lyrics and music as they relate to a child's life, fostering insight and self-reflection to connect emotions with experiences.

Music games are interactive activities that involve music, encouraging social interaction and engagement, helping build social skills, cooperation, and a sense of community. Performing gives children, the opportunity to express their thoughts and feelings in real-time through the re-creation of pre-composed songs or renditions of their compositions. In addition, combining visual arts with music provides an opportunity for expression through multiple modalities, encouraging creativity and self-expression while accommodating diverse learning styles.

Group music therapy involves a music therapist working with several individuals simultaneously. Music therapists engage small groups of individuals, often with similar needs or objectives in therapeutic music experiences. Group settings can provide opportunities for social interaction, peer support, and collective expression through music. This format allows participants to interact with others who may be experiencing similar issues, providing validation, support, and perspective. Group music therapy can be particularly effective for addressing specific concerns such as addiction, grief, trauma, or social skills development.

Community music therapy (CoMT), as we also will review in Chap. 3, focuses on promoting mental health and well-being within a specific community or population (Stige & Aarø, 2012). At this level, music therapy extends its reach beyond individual clients or groups to address the needs of a broader community. This could involve offering music therapy programmes in child protection institutions, schools or community centres, hospitals, or other local institutions to promote wellness and social cohesion.

While less commonly discussed, the principles of music therapy can also be applied to global challenges and initiatives, such as in the case with UNCRC (1989). For example, music can be used as a means of promoting cross-cultural understanding, fostering peacebuilding efforts, creating awareness of children's rights, or addressing global sustainability issues (Krüger, 2020). Technology has made it possible for music therapists to disseminate ways in which they use music-based experiences to support children's rights and address global issues. In this book we will highlight research from the international music therapy community, supporting the notion that music therapy is a global profession.

Child-Centred Music Therapy and Professional Discretion

The concept of discretion, a fundamental aspect of modern societies, has deep historical roots, as noted by Molander (2016). This idea can be traced back to Aristotle's *Nicomachean Ethics* (Ross & Brown, 2009, cited in Molander, 2016), where he distinguishes between three types of knowledge. Aristotle's framework of practical wisdom, or *phronesis*, plays a crucial role in understanding how discretion is exercised in moral and ethical decision-making. By exploring these types of knowledge, we gain insights into the complexities of discretion, which continues to shape human judgement and behaviour in contemporary society.

Episteme: Scientific, context-independent knowledge.

Techne: Craft knowledge based on practical rationality.

Phronesis: Practical wisdom, emphasizing reflection and its relationship to wise action (p. 35).

Polanyi (1967) expands on this by introducing the concept of tacit knowledge—understanding that is embedded in action but difficult to articulate, such as knowing how to ride a bike or swim. Schön (1983) builds on both Aristotle and Polanyi, focusing on the "epistemology of practice" in professions where uncertainty and conflict are present. He identifies three types of reflection:

Reflection-in-action: Reflecting while engaged in practice.

Reflection-on-action: Reflecting after the action to inform future decisions.

Reflection-in-practice: Ongoing reflection aimed at improving approaches (p. 31).

Tan et al. (2023) critique Schön's approach, arguing that reflection should not be confined to individual introspection but should also involve collaboration with colleagues. They advocate for teamwork and collective reflection, such as the "reflecting teams" concept in family therapy (Andersen, 1987). Following this, Lipsky (2010) defines discretion as the ability of professionals to make decisions based on their own judgement, a process where mistakes or arbitrary decisions can arise. While professional discretion can pose risks, it also provides room for autonomy and ethical decision-making. Inspired by this line of reasoning, we believe that professional discretion in music therapy involves the therapist's capacity to make thoughtful and context-sensitive decisions that prioritize the child's rights, well-being, and individual needs.

Based on the foregoing, we understand child-centred music therapy as an approach that through professional discretion integrates the principles of child rights into music therapy practices and research:

> Child-centred music therapy, in line with the United Nations Convention on the Rights of the Child (UNCRC), focuses on the child's individual needs, preferences, and rights throughout the therapeutic process. It upholds the UNCRC's principles by ensuring children have the right to actively participate in decisions that affect them (Article 12), express themselves freely (Article 13), and grow in a safe, supportive environment (Article 6). This approach empowers children to engage creatively and emotionally, placing them at the heart of their therapeutic experience.

This approach prioritizes the child's emotional, psychological, and developmental needs by ensuring that therapeutic interventions are tailored to the individual, their circumstances, preferences, and strengths. It emphasizes creating a safe, supportive environment where children can express themselves through music, fostering their creativity and resilience. In this context, practitioners actively involve the child in the therapeutic process, considering their opinions and feelings in decision-making. The focus is on enhancing the child's overall well-being and development while respecting their rights as outlined in the UNCRC (United Nations, 1989).

In a child-centred approach, as framed by the UNCRC, the exercise of discretion ensures that the child's voice is heard and respected within the therapeutic process. Music therapists must reflect *in-action*, *on-action*, and *in-practice*, not only to make informed decisions during sessions but also to continuously adapt their methods to the evolving needs of the child (Bruscia, 2015). This process emphasizes collaboration with the child and, where appropriate, with family members and other professionals, ensuring that decisions are made in the child's best interest, fostering autonomy and emotional growth within a supportive, rights-respecting environment. By involving the child in decision-making and using music as a means of self-expression and emotional development, the therapist's discretion becomes a tool for empowering the child, while ensuring that professional autonomy is exercised with ethical and reflective awareness. Music therapists should, therefore, be encouraged to exercise discretion in making nuanced clinical decisions. However, there is a lack of research on professional discretion within music therapy, especially regarding how, when, and why discretion about the child's best interests is applied.

Critique Against the Best Interest of the Child

Writing about children's rights and child-centred music therapy requires a critical examination of what these rights represent. The UNCRC (1989) does not provide a precise definition of the "best interests of the child," and one of the main critiques of this phrase is that it is vague and imprecise. While the term "best interests" broadly refers to a child's well-being, it is impossible to offer a definitive definition because it depends on various individual circumstances, such as the child's age and maturity, the presence or absence of parents, and the child's environment.

Tushnet (1992) argues that a rights discourse can obscure harsh realities within the law, such as oppression, greed, and self-interest. Those in power can manipulate the meaning of 'rights' because the concept is vague and indeterminate. The 'regime of rights,' he argues, can oppress society, with the rights discourse acting as a smokescreen, concealing more complex and challenging issues. As such, "rights-talk" from politicians or people with authorities may at times foster excessive individualism and lead to the neglect of responsibilities (Unger, 1986). Hunt (1990) expresses it this way:

> Rights have the capacity to be elements of emancipation, but they are neither a perfect nor exclusive vehicle for the emancipation. [They] can only be operative as constituents of a strategy for social transformation as they become part of an emergent "common sense" and are articulated with social practices. (p. 325)

Based on Hunt's definition, we can say that children's rights need to become integrated into the language and practices of music therapy to make a meaningful impact. In other words, the discourse of children's rights may become vague if not anchored in a specific context, such as music therapy. Moreover, children's rights can be criticized for being unrealistic, as they do not consider the economic, social, and political differences between countries (Unger, 1986). It is challenging to apply the same rights universally, given that children do not live under the same conditions globally. The ambiguity surrounding a child's best interests leaves room for manipulation. These arguments draw upon ideas central to the movement initiated by Arnstein (1969) and her concept of a Ladder of Participation. Arnstein's ideas, developed in the late 1960s, retain considerable relevance today, particularly in child welfare practice. At the top of the ladder, we find "Citizen Control," while at the lower steps lies "Nonparticipation." Interestingly, Arnstein categorizes "Therapy" alongside "Manipulation," creating space for paradoxical circumstances to arise.

A fundamental paradox within the concept of a child's best interests relates to viewing children as both dependent and independent (Krüger, 2020). Children should not be seen solely as strong and independent adults, but they are also not entirely helpless or in need of constant assistance. Instead, they should be regarded as competent individuals entitled to be heard and to influence matters concerning themselves (Langford et al., 2019). Additionally, the best interests of the child recognize children as active agents, capable of drawing on their resources and competencies (Jones et al., 2021).

A second paradox applies to the individual rights of the child. The UNCRC states that each child is unique and entitled to individual support and protection. However, the individual child must engage with local community cultures to fully realize these rights. Given the inherent dilemmas and paradoxes of the UNCRC (1989), the use of professional discretion and collaborative teamwork among professionals becomes essential in finding this balance.

The UNCRC advocates for a child's right to thrive in environments that respects their dignity, safety, and equality. In contexts where systemic discrimination exists, individual resilience alone is insufficient to overcome generational trauma and deprivation of socioeconomic opportunities. The UNCRC calls for a collective responsibility to address historical and ongoing human rights violations by dismantling systemic barriers that affect children's well-being and ensuring equal access to resources such as housing, education, and healthcare. Thus, while fostering individual resilience is essential, it must be coupled with structural reforms that address the root causes of inequality and injustice, ensuring that all children can grow and develop in fair and supportive environments.

References

Andersen, T. (1987). The reflecting team: Dialogue and meta-dialogue in clinical work. *Family Process, 26*(4), 415–428. https://doi.org/10.1111/j.1545-5300.1987.00415.x

Aristotle. (2015). *Politics* (C. D. C. Reeve, Trans.). Hackett Publishing Company.

Arnstein, S. R. (1969). A ladder of citizen participation. *Journal of the American Planning Association, 35*(4), 216–224.

Blacking, J. (1978). *How musical is man?* University of Washington Press.

Bruscia, K. E. (2015). *Reflexivity in music therapy: An anthology.* Barcelona Publishers.

Children and Families Act 2014, c.6. https://www.legislation.gov.uk/ukpga/2014/6/contents/enacted

Children, Youth and Family Services Act. 2017. S.O. 2017, c. 14, Sched. 1. Retrieved from https://www.ontario.ca/laws/statute/17c14

Curtis, S., & Vaillancourt, G. (2012). The children's right to music project. *Voices: A World Forum for Music Therapy, 12*(3).

Enge, K. E. A., & Stige, B. (2022). Musical pathways to the peer community: A collective case study of refugee children's use of music therapy. *Nordic Journal of Music Therapy, 31*(1), 7–24. https://doi.org/10.1080/08098131.2021.1891130

Eriksen, M. H. (2017). Don't all mothers love their children? Deposited infants as animate objects in the Scandinavian iron age. *World Archaeology, 49*(3), 338–356. https://doi.org/10.1080/00438243.2017.1340189

Fairchild, R., & Mraz, M. (2018). "Everything changed when I got those drums": A collaborative case reflection. *Voices: A World Forum for Music Therapy, 18*(1), 1–13. https://doi.org/10.15845/voices.v18i1.957

Fairchild, R., Thompson, G., & McFerran, K. S. (2017). Exploring the meaning of a performance in music therapy for children and their families experiencing homelessness and family violence. *Music Therapy Perspectives, 35*(1), 36–49. https://doi.org/10.1093/mtp/miw004

Falch-Eriksen, A., & Backe-Hansen, E. (2018). Child protection and human rights: A call for professional practice and policy. In A. Falch-Eriksen & E. Backe-Hansen (Eds.), *Human rights in child protection: Implications for professional practice* (pp. 1–15). Palgrave Macmillan.

Fancourt, D., & Finn, S. (2019). *What is the evidence on the role of the arts in improving health and wellbeing? A scoping review* (Health Evidence Network synthesis report, 6). World Health Organization Regional Office for Europe. https://www.euro.who.int/en/publications/abstracts/what-is-the-evidence-on-the-role-of-the-arts-in-improving-health-and-well-being-a-scoping-review-2019

Hakomäki, H. (2012). Storycomposing as a method in music therapy. A collaborative experiment with a young co-researcher. In G. Trondalen & K. Stensæth (Eds.), *Barn, musikk, helse* (Vol. 3). Series from Centre for Research in Music and Health (CREMAH).

Helle-Valle, A. (2016). *How do we understand children's restlessness? A cooperative and reflexive exploration of children's restlessness as a bioecological phenomenon* (Doctoral dissertation). University of Bergen.

Hindle, S. (2000). *The state and social change in early modern England*. Palgrave Macmillan.

Hunt, A. (1990). Rights and social movements: Counter-hegemonic strategies. *Journal of Law and Society, 17*(3), 309–328.

Jebb, E. (1924). *Declaration of the rights of the child*. League of Nations.

Jones, G. (2002). *Killing infants: Angel makers in Europe from the 19th to 20th centuries*. Oxford University Press.

Jones, P., Cedar, L., Coleman, A., Haythorne, D., Mercieca, D., & Ramsden, E. (2021). *Child agency and voice in therapy: New ways of working in the arts therapies*. Routledge.

Kilday, A. M., & Nash, D. (2023). 'Angels of the House' or 'Angel-Makers'? Problematizing murderous mothers in the nineteenth century. *Beyond deviant damsels: Re-evaluating female criminality in the nineteenth century* (Oxford, 2023; online edn, Oxford Academic, March 23, 2023). Retrieved October 1, 2024, from https://doi.org/10.1093/oso/9780198830733.003.0004.

Klyve, G. P., & Rolvsjord, R. (2022). Moments of fun: Narratives of children's experiences of music therapy in mental health care. *Nordic Journal of Music Therapy, 32*(2), 100–120. https://doi.org/10.1080/08098131.2022.2055114

Krüger, V. (2020). *Music therapy in child welfare: Bridging provision, protection, and participation*. Barcelona Publishers.

Langford, M., Skivenes, M., Søvig, K. H., & Loven Kirkebø, T. (2019). Introduction: Implementing child rights. In M. Langford, M. Skivenes, & K. H. Søvig (Eds.), *Children's rights in Norway: An implementation paradox?* (pp. 15–41). Universitetsforlaget.

Lansdown, G. (2011). *Every child's right to be heard: A resource guide on the UN Committee on the Rights of the Child General Comment No.12*. Save the Children/UNICEF.

Lipsky, M. (2010). *Street-level bureaucracy. Dilemmas of the individual in public services* (30th Anniversary Expanded ed.). Russel Sage Foundation.

Metell, M. (2023). *Disabled children's access to music*. Music's Transform.

Mitchell, E. (2023). Music's relational imperative: Wellbeing, music-making, and the interconnections between music therapy and music education. In K. S. Hendricks (Ed.), *The Oxford handbook of care in music education* (pp. 361–372). Oxford University Press. https://doi.org/10.1093/oxfordhb/9780197611654.013.33

Molander, A. (2016). *Discretion in the welfare state: Social rights and professional judgment*. Routledge.

Oranga Tamariki Act. 1989/2019, No 24 (as amended in 2019). Retrieved from https://www.legislation.govt.nz/act/public/1989/0024/latest/DLM147088.html

Oselame, M. do N. (2023). "*No não sentir não há sentido": A musicoterapia como uma prática de cuidado em saúde no sistema socioeducativo* (Doctoral thesis). Fundação Oswaldo Cruz—Escola Nacional de Saúde Pública Sergio Arouca.

Polanyi, M. (1967). *The tacit dimension* (Vol. A540, pp. xi, 108). Doubleday.

Ross, W. D., & Brown, L. (2009). *The Nicomachean ethics*. Oxford University Press.

Schön, D. A. (1983). *The reflective practitioner: How professionals think in action*. Basic Books.

Simensen, E. (Ed.). (2021). *The older Gulathing law* (1st ed., Chapter 21). Routledge.

Skivenes, M., & Sørsdal, L. M. (2018). The child's best interest principle across child protection jurisdictions. In A. Falch-Eriksen & E. Backe-Hansen (Eds.), *Human rights in child protection* (pp. 59–88). Palgrave Macmillan. https://doi.org/10.1007/978-3-319-94800-3_4

Small, C. (1998). *Musicking: The meanings of performing and listening*. Wesleyan University Press.

Stige, B., & Aarø, L. E. (2012). *Invitation to community music therapy*. Routledge.

Tan, L., Kocsis, A., & Burry, J. (2023). Advancing Donald Schön's reflective practitioner: Where to next? *Design Issues, 39*(3), 3–18. https://doi.org/10.1162/desi_a_00722

Trehub, S. E., Becker, J., & Morley, I. (2015). Cross-cultural perspectives on music and musicality. *Philosophical Transactions of the Royal Society of London. Series B, Biological Sciences, 370*(1664), 20140096. https://doi.org/10.1098/rstb.2014.0096

Tushnet, M. (1992). The critique of rights. *Southern Methodist University Law Review, 47*, 23–34.

UN Committee on the Rights of the Child (UNCRC). (2013). *General comment No. 14 on the right of the child to have his or her best interests taken as a primary consideration (art. 3, para. 1)*. CRC/C/GC/14. Retrieved from https://www2.ohchr.org/english/bodies/crc/docs/gc/crc_c_gc_14_eng.pdf

Unger, R. M. (1986). *The critical legal studies movement*. Harvard University Press.

United Nations. (1989). *Convention on the rights of the child*. https://www.ohchr.org/en/instruments-mechanisms/instruments/convention-rights-child

United Nations General Assembly. (1959). *Declaration of the Rights of the Child*. Retrieved from https://digitallibrary.un.org/record/195831?ln=en&v=pdf

Victorian Government, Department of Health and Human Services. (2018). *Home Stretch Program*. Retrieved from https://www.vic.gov.au/home stretch

CHAPTER 2

Integrating and Weighing the Elements of the Best Interests of the Child in Music Therapy Practice

Elements to be considered when assessing the child's best interests (GC No. 14, 2013).

(a) The child's views
(b) The child's identity (and culture)
(c) Preservation of the family environment and maintaining relations
(d) Care, protection and safety of the child
(e) Situation of vulnerability
(f) The child's right to health
(g) The child's right to education

Introduction

In this chapter we review how music therapy can support a best interest's assessment. The Committee on the Rights of the Child published a document aimed at addressing the lack of a common understanding of the "best interest principle" (GC No. 14, 2013). Part V of this comment outlines seven elements that should be considered when a decision about the child's best interests is to be made including (a) the child's views; (b) the child's identity; (c) preservation of the family environment and maintaining relations; (d) care, protection, and safety of the child; (e)

V. Krüger, K. M. Murphy, *Child-Centred Music Therapy*,
https://doi.org/10.1007/978-3-031-85724-9_2

evaluation of vulnerability; (f) the child's right to health, and (g) the child's right to education. To weigh the elements against each other, a best interest of the child depends on collaboration with an interdisciplinary team.

In the chapter we will highlight music therapy's potential to contribute in interdisciplinary settings. We believe we can meet the "best interest of the child" principle through collaboration with other professionals, agencies, families, and stakeholders.

The Child's Own View

Article 12 of the Convention provides for the right of children to express their views in every decision that affects them. Any decision that does not consider the child's views or does not give their views due weight according to their age and maturity does not respect the possibility for the child or children to influence the determination of their best interests.

The fact that the child is very young or in a vulnerable situation (e.g. has a disability, belongs to a minority group, is a migrant, etc.) does not deprive him or her of the right to express his or her views, nor reduces the weight given to the child's views in determining his or her best interests. The adoption of specific measures to guarantee the exercise of equal rights for children in such situations must be subject to an individual assessment which assures a role to the children themselves in the decision-making process, and the provision of reasonable accommodation[9] and support, where necessary, to ensure their full participation in the assessment of their best interests (GC No. 14, 2013).

Music therapy is highly relevant to Article 12 of the Convention, which emphasizes the child's right to express their views in decisions affecting them. Participation in music therapy provides children, including those who are young or in vulnerable situations, the opportunity to express their thoughts and emotions non-verbally, providing a means of communication for those who struggle to express themselves through words. Music therapy often provides a supportive space where children's voices are heard and respected, ensuring that their views are given due consideration in decisions regarding their well-being and best interests.

There is a growing body of literature in music therapy that stresses the importance of child's view (e.g. Krüger et al., 2023). Participants in music therapy themselves are best for illustrating how music therapy may facilitate a safe space where, for example, they can express frustration:

> When you live in an institution, there's always a lot going through your mind. You're always thinking about a lot of things: moving home, where you're going to be, what you want to do, who you want to be with. And when I've come here [to the music therapy workshop], I've been able to "cleanse" and express that frustration. Every time I've done that; it's made things better and better. (Krüger, 2020, p. 19)

The Lundy model supports an approach to music therapy that ensures that children's voices are heard, and their rights respected (see Fairchild et al., 2017). The model identifies four key elements of the right to be heard:

Space: Children need to have a safe and supportive space to express their views. This could be a physical space, such as a meeting room, a music room, or a playroom, or it could be a metaphorical space, such as a time and place where children feel comfortable talking about their experiences.

Voice: Children need to be able to express their views in a way that is understandable to the adults who are listening. This could involve using music, words, drawings, or other forms of communication.

Audience: Children need to have someone who is willing to listen to their views and take them seriously. This could be a parent, music therapist, teacher, social worker, or other adult who is responsible for making decisions about the child's life.

Influence: Children's views need to have a real impact on the decisions that are made about them. This means that adults need to be willing to take children's views into account and to make changes to their decisions if necessary (Lundy et al., 2011).

The model has been used to involve children in decision-making about their schooling (Klyve & Rolvsjord, 2022), and in child protection determinations (Krüger, 2020). Further, it justifies children's involvement in decisions about their health care including giving them the opportunity to meet with doctors and nurses, to express their views about their treatment, and to make decisions about their own care. Listening to the voice of the child involves balancing the child's perspective and needs with the views of others. Any decision that does not consider the child's views or does not give their views due weight according to their age and maturity, does not allow children the option to influence the determination of their best interests. The fact that the child is very young or in a vulnerable situation (has a disability, belongs to a minority group, is a migrant, etc.) should not deprive them of the right to express their views nor reduce the weight given to the child's views in determining their best interests.

The Lundy model is closely connected to the right to participation, a concept explained by Brodie et al. (2009) and applied in music therapy research (e.g. Krüger et al., 2023). Firstly, participation should be understood from the perspective of those who are participating, implying that participation is rooted in the participant's experience. Therefore, therapeutic efforts must commence with an understanding of the young person's emotional life, relationships, and their genuine interest in involvement. Establishing trust therefore is a prerequisite for successful participation. The second factor is that participation occurs within a contextualized practice. Professionals working with children across the disciplines must understand the child's sociocultural background to facilitate their involvement in participation processes. In music therapy, this may involve familiarizing oneself with the child's musical preferences, as well as aspects such as gender, nationality, or cultural background. The third factor is relationships, both interpersonal and contextual. Music therapists should consider genuine participation as requisite for the establishment of a connection between how children/young people engage with music in everyday situations and structured activities led by adults, such as informal cultural school programmes, bands, or choirs (Krüger, 2016). The fourth factor concerns power. Participation requires an analysis of who has power to define practice, and a willingness to allow a certain transfer of power. Overall, participation is a contextualized phenomenon. That is, participation experience is built on knowledge of the qualities and aspects of how people relate to each other in different situations and social networks. Music therapy supports agents in revealing power structures and facilitates dialogues that promote voice and agency (Jones et al., 2021).

The Child's Identity

Children are not a homogeneous group and therefore diversity must be taken into account when assessing their best interests. The identity of the child includes characteristics such as sex, sexual orientation, national origin, religion and beliefs, cultural identity, personality. Although children and young people share basic universal needs, the expression of those needs depends on a wide range of personal, physical, social, and cultural aspects, including their evolving capacities. The right of the child to preserve his or her identity is guaranteed by the Convention (Article 8) and must be respected and taken into consideration in the assessment of the child's best interests.

Regarding religious and cultural identity, for example, when considering a foster home or placement for a child, due regard shall be paid to the desirability of continuity in a child's upbringing and to the child's ethnic, religious, cultural, and linguistic background (Article 20, para. 3), and the decision-maker must take into consideration this specific context when assessing and determining the child's best interests. The same applies in cases of adoption, separation from or divorce of parents. Due consideration of the child's best interests implies that children have access to the culture (and language, if possible) of their country and family of origin, and the opportunity to access information about their biological family, in accordance with the legal and professional regulations of the given country (see Article 9, para. 4).

Although preservation of religious and cultural values and traditions as part of the identity of the child must be taken into consideration, practices that are inconsistent or incompatible with the rights established in the Convention are not in the child's best interests. Cultural identity cannot excuse or justify the perpetuation by decision-makers and authorities of traditions and cultural values that deny the child or children the rights guaranteed by the Convention (GC No. 14, 2013).

Music therapy allows for understanding children's diverse identities, as it provides a flexible and culturally sensitive approach to support their emotional and social development. By incorporating elements of a child's cultural, religious, and personal background into therapeutic practices, music therapists can help preserve their identity while meeting their unique emotional and developmental needs. For children in foster care, waiting for adoption, or similar vulnerable situations, music therapy can offer a creative means to express their cultural heritage, maintain a sense of continuity in their upbringing, and strengthen their evolving capacities, all while ensuring that their rights under the Convention are respected.

In general, assessing identity concerns the right to preserve nationality, name, and family relations. However, when read in conjunction with the rest of the Convention, the right to identity can be understood in relation to other aspects of children's identity, such as their sexual orientation and the right to their own culture, with a particular awareness of aspects related to cultural sensitivity and otherness. The theme of identity is central to music therapy. Young people use music as a resource for agency and empowerment in identity construction processes (Saarikallio, 2019). Music is involved in the way young people construct their own self-image and strengthen their self-esteem (Beckmann, 2013). Participation in music therapy may empower children to express their cultural identity (Derrington, 2019; Krüger & Tuastad, 2025).

The view that participation in music therapy can develop and support identity can partly be traced back to Ruud (2010). According to Ruud, music can provide a person with identity formatting resources, including gender, social class, or ethnic background. The music becomes markers of important transitions and junctions in life, like a soundtrack in life (Bruscia, 1998; Ruud, 2010). The music can mark transitions from one phase of life to another, like movements through liminal phases (Ruud, 1998). Ruud also describes the transpersonal space. That music accompanies people throughout their life, including transitions between situations and events, is an understanding that is especially significant for those of us who work with children and young people. Music may help some with transitions through various life stages from childhood until the end of life.

Cultural Sensitivity

Cultural sensitivity refers to decision-makers' awareness and appreciation of children's ethnicity, language, religion, nationality, or migrant background and should be considered in music therapy practice. Music, as a culturally embedded phenomenon, both shapes and is shaped by culture (Baines, 2013). It holds a significant role in social settings, and the meaning of a musical experience is often influenced by the listener's cultural background and personal context (Chase, 2004). In a position paper Mahoney (2015) explains this involves understanding how a child's culture(s) may influence their approach to participation and communication. Several music therapy scholars (e.g. Bruscia, 2015; dos Santos, 2024) emphasize the importance of a reflexive approach, urging therapists to develop cross-cultural awareness in two key areas.

According to Ruud (1998), music therapists should "have a musical cultural understanding, a deep respect for the individual or idiosyncratic and sometimes subcultural representation of music" (p. 25). There is a risk in perceiving music as a universal language, recognized and accessible to all, as it may create the false notion that multicultural considerations are not necessarily an issue in music therapy (Brown, 2002). Pavlicevic (2003) notes that music therapists must be sensitive to the cultural, social, and musical norms and "[...] be informed and sensitive when selecting music for sessions. For many cultural groups there may be religious or cultural associations (and sensitivities) around certain music" (p. 67).

Scrine (2019) argues that music therapists play a crucial role in challenging and reframing discourses that marginalize or overly victimize young people based on their gender and sexuality. Their writings highlight how contemporary music therapy practices can move beyond traditional views by fostering collaboration with young people, addressing oppressive norms, and engaging in social action. To support the well-being and development of adolescents, it is essential for therapists to critically examine fixed notions of gender and sexuality and understand how these intersect with factors like race, culture, and class. By recognizing and addressing these structures of oppression, music therapy can serve as a powerful intervention, not only within the therapeutic space but also in broader societal contexts. This approach allows for a more nuanced understanding of how norms and their impacts vary among individuals, thereby promoting a more inclusive and equitable practice.

It is essential that music therapists have an openness to explore their own cultural identity, as well as the identity of the child (Donley, 2020) as cultural assumptions, cultural values, misinterpretation, and culturally unsuitable reactions can occur in the therapeutic process. Therefore, an awareness of the patient's cultural world is critical (Bell, 2016). Music therapists must explore personal biases related to cultural differences in general and more specifically to the patient's cultural background (Gonzalez, 2011). Both perspectives of cultural consideration—the music therapist's self-exploration and the understanding of the patient's culture—are essential, and differences and similarities that exist between the music therapist and the patient need to be taken into consideration as this may affect the therapeutic process (Hadley & Norris, 2016). Music is a process based on elusive cultural symbols that contain meanings beyond verbal definitions and is a fundamental element of the cultural experience (Gouk, 2017). It is recommended that music therapists practice cultural humility while assessing the best interest of the child as it helps to build trust with the child and their family. This involves active listening, showing respect, and demonstrating cultural sensitivity in interactions. It also involves collaboration with the child, their family, and other relevant professionals, helping to ensure that decisions are made that are culturally appropriate and in the best interests of the child.

Preservation of the Family Environment and Maintaining Relations

The term "family" must be interpreted in a broad sense to include biological, adoptive, or foster parents or, where applicable, the members of the extended family or community as provided for by local custom (Article 5). Preventing family separation and preserving family unity are important components of the child protection system and are based on the right provided for in Article 9, paragraph 1, which requires "that a child shall not be separated from his or her parents against their will, except when [...] such separation is

(*continued*)

(continued)

necessary for the best interests of the child." Furthermore, the child who is separated from one or both parents is entitled "to maintain personal relations and direct contact with both parents on a regular basis, except if it is contrary to the child's best interests" (Article 9, para. 3). This also extends to any person holding custody rights, legal or customary primary caregivers, foster parents, and persons with whom the child has a strong personal relationship. Given the gravity of the impact on the child of separation from his or her parents, such separation should only occur as a last resort measure, as when the child is in danger of experiencing imminent harm or when otherwise necessary; separation should not take place if less intrusive measures could protect the child. Before resorting to separation, the State should provide support to the parents in assuming their parental responsibilities and restore or enhance the family's capacity to take care of the child, unless separation is necessary to protect the child. Economic reasons cannot be a justification for separating a child from his or her parents (GC No. 14, 2013).

There is a growing body of literature that supports music therapy as a means of promoting family connection. Music therapy is particularly relevant in a family setting because it can help strengthen relationships, foster emotional connections, and support the overall well-being of children and their caregivers (Cotter & Krüger, in press). Given the emphasis on preserving family unity, as described in the UNCRC, music therapy offers a supportive approach that promotes communication, bonding, and promotion of participation (Jacobsen, 2019). Music therapy can be especially useful in situations where a child is at risk of separation or has experienced trauma, as it helps to maintain strong personal relations and address emotional needs within the family unit, thereby reducing the need for separation (Sutton, 2002). Music therapy can provide an alternative to traditional talk therapy, especially because it helps adults to establish contact with children and adolescents (Bolger, 2013; Hussey et al., 2007). Music therapy can help to promote an environment that creates well-being and happiness, for example, in school or institutional contexts as young people frequently engage in music experiences (Rickson & McFerran, 2014; McFerran & Teggelove, 2011). However, in weighing the different interests of the child, protection from unnecessary pressure and privacy intrusions can become crucial when involving children in music therapy.

Care, Protection, and Safety of the Child

When assessing and determining the best interests of a child or children in general, the obligation of the State to ensure the child such protection and care as is necessary for his or her well-being (Article 3, para. 2) should be taken into consideration. The terms "protection and care" must also be read in a broad sense, since their objective is not stated in limited or negative terms (such as "to protect the child from harm"), but rather in relation to the comprehensive ideal of ensuring the child's "well-being" and development.

Children's well-being, in a broad sense includes their basic material, physical, educational, and emotional needs, as well as needs for affection and safety.

Emotional care is a basic need of children; if parents or other primary caregivers do not fulfil the child's emotional needs, action must be taken so that the child develops a secure attachment. Children need to form an attachment to a caregiver at a very early age, and such attachment, if adequate, must be sustained over time to provide the child with a stable environment.

Assessment of the child's best interests must also include consideration of the child's safety, that is, the right of the child to protection against all forms of physical or mental violence, injury or abuse (Article 19), sexual harassment, peer pressure, bullying, degrading treatment, and so on (Article 14) as well as protection against sexual, economic, and other exploitations, drugs, labour, armed conflict, and so on (Articles 32–39).

Applying a best-interests approach to decision-making means assessing the safety and integrity of the child at the current time; however, the precautionary principle also requires assessing the possibility of future risk and harm and other consequences of the decision for the child's safety (GC No. 14, 2013).

Music therapy plays an essential role in supporting the well-being and emotional care of children which are critical aspects of determining their best interests. By offering a therapeutic environment where children can express emotions, develop trust, and build secure attachments, music therapy addresses their emotional and psychological needs. This aligns with the comprehensive approach to child protection that emphasizes not only safeguarding children from harm but also ensuring their emotional development and secure attachment to caregivers. Music therapy can be valuable for nurturing emotional safety and resilience, which are key elements in creating a stable environment for the child's well-being.

Themes

such as care, protection, and safety are prominent in music therapy literature (Trondalen, 2016; Zanders, 2015). A safe relationship with the music therapist can help children and young people to develop self-esteem in the face of other children and adults. Rolvsjord (2010) proposes that music therapy provides opportunities and possibilities for voicing negative emotions and trauma. Music therapy methods such as songwriting (Fairchild & McFerran, 2019) and improvisation (Ruud, 1998) may provide confirmation, recognition, and an understanding of difficult emotions. Expressing emotions in general can be a huge challenge in and of itself for many who have been traumatized (van der Kolk, 2014). The process of using music therapy in this way may facilitate tolerance and expression of uncomfortable emotions. Further, these difficult emotions can be processed within a safe container created by the music and trusting relationship with the therapist (de Baker, 1993).

Music therapy can also bring into focus the relationship between strengths and needs, as it does with resources and problems. The interaction in music therapy can allow the child to be both strong and weak, that is, to encounter ambivalence connected to acknowledging one's own strengths (Rolvsjord, 2010, p. 168). Safety provided during music therapy sessions may serve as a springboard to help children get in contact with their own feelings (Johns, 2017). Music therapy may help to expand the child's window of tolerance (Siegel, 2012), which is a goal for trauma therapy. The "window of tolerance" is a concept developed by Siegel that describes the optimal zone of arousal in which an individual can effectively process information and engage with their environment. Within this window, a person can manage emotions and reactions, allowing for adaptive functioning in social, emotional, and cognitive domains. When a person experiences either hyperarousal (intense emotional states such as anxiety or panic) or hypoarousal (dissociation or numbness), they move outside this window, leading to difficulties in emotional regulation and interpersonal relationships (Siegel, 2012). In the context of music therapy, the window of tolerance is particularly relevant. Music therapists often aim to create a safe and supportive environment that enables clients to explore their emotions and experiences without exceeding their window of tolerance. Music can serve as a powerful tool to help children stay within this optimal zone, facilitating emotional expression and regulation. For instance, engaging with music can evoke feelings that allow individuals to reconnect with their emotions in a manageable way, promoting healing and growth.

Situation of Vulnerability

An important element to consider is the child's situation of vulnerability, such as disability, belonging to a minority group, being a refugee or asylum seeker, victim of abuse, and living in a street situation. The purpose of determining the best interests of a child or children in a vulnerable situation should not only be in relation to the full enjoyment of all the rights provided for in the Convention, but also with regard to other human rights norms related to these specific situations, such as those covered in the Convention on the Rights of Persons with Disabilities and the Convention relating to the Status of Refugees.

The best interests of a child in a specific situation of vulnerability will not be the same as those of all the children in the same vulnerable situation. Authorities and decision-makers need to consider the different kinds and degrees of vulnerability of each child, as each child is unique, and each situation must be assessed according to the child's uniqueness. An individualized assessment of each child's history from birth should be carried out, with regular reviews by a multidisciplinary team and recommended reasonable accommodation throughout the child's development process (GC No. 14, 2013).

Music therapy is especially relevant for children in vulnerable situations, such as those with disabilities, refugees, or victims of abuse, as it offers a personalized and supportive way to address their emotional and psychological needs. By using music in therapy, children can safely express their emotions, foster resilience, and build connections in ways that are adapted to their unique experiences and vulnerabilities. Music therapy's flexible and individualized approach aligns with the need for tailored interventions that consider each child's specific circumstances, helping to promote healing and well-being in a safe and nurturing environment.

Music therapists working with children who live in vulnerable situations need to take into consideration that their efforts may be disempowering. Music therapists are in the position of power and can contribute to structures that can lead to sense of disempowerment. This power structure may lead to paternalism on the part of the therapist. The concept of paternalism refers to the practice of making decisions on behalf of others without considering their perspectives, needs, or desires (Knijn & van Nijnatten, 2011). This can take many forms, including the imposition of certain identities, the control of a social situation, or the limitation of verbal or nonverbal expression. Paternalistic decision-making can result in the suppression of creativity and the marginalization of certain individuals or communities. To avoid negative aspects of paternalism, it is important to promote an inclusive and democratic approach to decision-making, where all stakeholders, including children, have a voice in shaping the direction of the service and practice. This involves promoting diversity and representation, supporting independent and alternative voices, and encouraging open and inclusive dialogue and engagement among all parties involved.

Paternalism can take the form of parents or other authority figures making decisions for children without considering their input or opinions. In most cases paternalism can have negative effects on children, as it can limit their agency and autonomy and undermine their sense of self-worth and confidence. Children who experience paternalism may be more likely to internalize harmful beliefs about their own capabilities and worth and may struggle to assert themselves and make decisions on their own later in life (Langford et al., 2019).

In the context of music therapy, paternalism would refer to the practice of imposing one's own judgements or preferences onto clients or patients, often without their full consent or input, under the belief that it is for their own good or well-being. A child-centred approach in music therapy, however, would involve providing opportunities for children to explore, experiment with, and create music on their own terms, rather than imposing a particular musical style or genre. This involves using a variety of musical materials, instruments, and technology to support children's musical learning and expression. Conversely, music therapists may reject a paternalistic approach, offering children a platform for expressing thoughts and emotions that may be difficult to articulate in conventional ways. Music therapists can give children the means to communicate on their terms, fostering their sense of agency. This participatory process not only validates children's experiences but also actively involves them in shaping therapeutic and societal decisions that affect their lives. In doing so, music therapists challenge adult-centred control, offering a model where children are seen not as recipients of care, but as contributors to solutions. When integrated into broader participatory frameworks, music therapy supports children's involvement in processes that shape their communities, ensuring their voices are heard and respected. By incorporating creative expression into participatory models, we not only enhance children's capacity to hold systems accountable but also promote more inclusive, transparent, and child-centred governance.

Health

> The child's right to health (Article 24) and his or her health condition are central in assessing the child's best interest. However, if there is more than one possible treatment for a health condition or if the outcome of a treatment is uncertain, the advantages of all possible treatments must be weighed against all possible risks and side effects, and the views of the child must also be given due weight based on his or her age and maturity. In this respect, children should be provided with adequate and appropriate information to understand the situation and all the relevant aspects in relation to their interests, and be allowed, when possible, to give their consent in an informed manner (GC No. 14, 2013).

Music therapy aligns with the child's right to health by offering a holistic treatment option that supports emotional, psychological, and social well-being, particularly in cases where medical outcomes are uncertain or multiple treatment options exist. It provides children with an integrative or complementary means of expressing their emotions, helping them cope with health challenges in a way that respects their maturity and individual preferences. By engaging children in the therapeutic process, music therapists help them to better understand their health situation and participate in decisions about their care, fostering informed consent and self-empowerment in alignment with Article 24 of the UNCRC.

The child's right to health (Article 24) includes central elements in assessing the child's best interest. In music therapy literature health is often described with performative qualities (e.g. Stige, 2002). Links between music and health are found within investigations of music and identity (MacDonald et al., 2013), and music and communication (Miell et al., 2005). DeNora (2007) considers the idea of health as performance:

> Health is performed in social settings and in relation to performance conventions and materials. When we have received a good 'report card' time and time again, we accumulate an identity—we are 'healthy'. (p. 272)

Following this line of reasoning, health musicking could be defined as the appraisal and appropriation of the health affordances of the arena, agenda, agents, activities, and artefacts of a music practice (Stige, 2002, p. 211). As such, health musicking is a concept that integrates music into the promotion and maintenance of health. A health musicking approach recognizes the therapeutic potential of music to enhance physical, emotional, and psychological well-being. Health musicking is a concept coined to embrace emotional expression and social connection and empower children by involving them actively in their recovery process. Consequently, health musicking fosters a holistic approach to child health care, ensuring that every child's developmental, emotional, and cultural needs are met.

Education

It is in the best interests of the child to have access to quality education, including early childhood education, non-formal or informal education and related activities, free of charge. All decisions on measures and actions concerning a specific child or a group of children must respect the best interests of the child or children, about education. In order to promote education, or better quality education, for more children, States parties need to have well-trained teachers and other professionals working in different education related settings, as well as a child-friendly environment and appropriate teaching and learning methods, taking into consideration that education is not only an investment in the future, but also an opportunity for joyful activities, respect, participation and fulfilment of ambitions. Responding to this requirement and enhancing children's responsibilities to overcome the limitations of their vulnerability of any kind will be in their best interests (GC No. 14, 2013).

Music therapy is intrinsically linked to the best interests of the child within the framework of quality education. It is in the best interests of the child to have access to quality education, including early childhood education, non-formal or informal education and related activities, free of charge. In recent years, there is growing interest the use of music as a resource in education. Such interest has gone beyond the more traditional modes of music education, and an increasing number of studies have explored the relationship between music, young people, and well-being. Many of these studies conducted in an education setting shown positive outcomes such as enhanced social functioning (Teachout, 2005), improved emotion regulation (Uhlig et al., 2018), better self-esteem (Costa-Giomi, 2004), violence prevention (Fairchild & Sheridan, 2018; Nöcker-Ribaupierre & Wölfl, 2010), increased coping skills, cooperation, and school engagement (Gill & Rickard, 2012; Krüger et al., 2019).

Uhlig et al. (2018) investigated the impact of a rhythm and poetry music therapy intervention on adolescent emotional self-regulation in a school setting. The music therapy group showed a significant effect on measures related to emotion regulation when compared to a control condition. Gold et al. (2017) compared in-school group music therapy to self-directed music listening activities. While both showed small improvement over time, there was no significant difference in effect between the two. Cobbett (2016), set out to provide educators with clearer evidence for how music therapy, can help engage hard-to-reach adolescents. In their study, 52 adolescents received music therapy while 29 did not. Both students' self-rated scores and staff-rated scores showed a significant improvement in the group who received music therapy, compared to the control group. Caló et al. (2020) examined the impact of a community-based music intervention for young people's well-being, and Haering (2022) explored how music therapy might enhance language skills and inclusion in multilingual classrooms, underscoring the potential effects of music therapy on children in multicultural school environments, focusing the dynamics of music therapy among children with language difficulties. In sum these studies suggest that children who received music therapy gained improvements in self-confidence, well-being, learning and engagement because of their participation in the school's music programmes.

Best Interest Determination (BID)

The case of ten-year-old Maya, a refugee separated from her family, illustrates the careful balance of protection and cultural continuity in the Best Interests Determination (BID) process. Maya's desire for family reunification was central, with her views expressed through drawings and conversations.

In the case of ten-year-old Maya, a refugee separated from her family during conflict, the Best Interests Determination (BID) process was initiated to ensure her well-being. Maya expressed a strong desire to reunite with her extended family, and her views were carefully

(*continued*)

(continued)
considered using age-appropriate methods, such as conversations through drawings and discussions about her hopes. Her cultural and linguistic identities were prioritized, and efforts were made to place her in a community where she could maintain her native language and traditions. The BID team located her aunt in a neighbouring country but concerns about the aunt's unstable living situation delayed immediate reunification. To ensure Maya's safety, she was placed in foster care while her aunt's circumstances were assessed. Recognizing Maya's vulnerability due to the trauma she experienced during her displacement, mental health support was provided, including counselling and music therapy, *which helped her express and process her emotions in a non-verbal, creative way. Music therapy sessions allowed Maya to connect with her cultural roots through familiar songs, giving her a sense of continuity and comfort amidst the upheaval. Additionally, her physical health was addressed through medical assessments, and she was enrolled in school with language support to help her integrate while continuing to teach her native tongue. Over time, after improving her aunt's living conditions, Maya was safely reunited with her family, balancing her need for protection with her desire for familial connection, and supporting her overall emotional and educational development.*[1]

The above vignette illustrates the need for taking many aspects of the child's environment into consideration when determining what's in the best interest of the child. The vignette highlights how music therapy interventions, including group participation, songwriting, and playlist creation, helped Maya build confidence, manage emotions, and gradually transition into mainstream educational settings while also addressing deeper mental health needs. BID is a principle enshrined in the United Nations Convention on the Rights of the Child (UNCRC), which mandates that

[1]This is a constructed case and bears no resemblance with any real person or circumstance.

the best interests of the child should be a primary consideration in all actions concerning children. The “best-interests assessment” evaluates all factors needed to decide what serves a specific child or group of children in a given situation, involving decision-makers, their staff—ideally a professional team—and the child’s participation (UNHCR, 2008). The “best-interests determination” is the formal process, with strict safeguards, that uses this assessment to identify the child’s best interests (GC No. 14, 2013).

This process involves evaluating various factors, including the child’s physical, emotional, social, and educational needs, to make informed decisions that promote their well-being and development. BID is designed to ensure that the child’s rights are safeguarded and promoted, and it plays a critical role in areas such as child protection, family law, education, healthcare, and social services (Lundy, 2007). BID is not a simple or singular decision but rather a complex and multidimensional process that involves the evaluation of various factors including the child’s physical, emotional, social, and educational needs. The decision-making process requires a thorough consideration of each child’s circumstances and the participation of multiple stakeholders including professionals from social work, psychology, law, health, and education sectors to form a holistic view of what is truly in the child’s best interest (Lansdown, 2011). Particularly important in the BID process is the child’s right to participation, as outlined in Article 12 of the UNCRC. This article emphasizes that children have the right to express their views freely in all matters affecting them and that those views must be given due weight in accordance with the child’s age and maturity. In practice, this means that a child should be actively involved in the BID process whenever possible, whether by directly expressing their preferences or by providing insight into their experiences and needs through appropriate channels (Archard & Skivenes, 2009).

Implementing Best Interests Determination involves carefully balancing several factors to ensure the child’s well-being. First, the child’s views must be actively considered, such as through age-appropriate interviews or creative activities like drawing to understand their feelings and preferences. For example, a child expressing a desire to stay with their biological family must be taken seriously, but this preference may need to be balanced against their safety if there’s a history of abuse. The child’s identity, including their cultural, linguistic, and religious background, should be respected. For instance, placing a child from a minority culture with a foster family that shares their cultural heritage can help preserve their sense of belonging. Maintaining family relationships, when safe, is also critical. If a child cannot live with their parents, ongoing contact with extended family may be arranged to maintain family ties. However, safety and protection must always be prioritized. For example, a child in a dangerous home environment may be removed, even if they wish to remain.

Children who are particularly vulnerable, such as those with disabilities or traumatic backgrounds, may require specialized care, like placement in homes with trained caregivers. Health needs, both physical and mental, must be addressed, such as ensuring access to medical care and counselling for a child with a history of neglect. Finally, education is crucial; for example, enrolling a displaced child in a local school ensures they have stability and opportunities for development. These elements often involve trade-offs, requiring a holistic approach where professionals weigh each factor to make decisions in the child's best interests.

Challenges with Music Therapy and BID

Following the line of reasoning presented in our book, in music therapy settings with children and adolescents, BID presents various challenges that can impede effective collaboration among diverse professionals and cultural groups, emphasizing the need for cultural competence and sensitivity. Acknowledging the distinct norms, values, and communication styles inherent to each discipline and cultural background is crucial for fostering inclusive therapeutic environments. For example, music therapists must be attuned to how cultural beliefs influence clients' relationships with music and therapy, as failing to recognize these differences can lead to tokenism and superficial integration of perspectives (e.g. Scrine, 2019). Additionally, communication barriers, such as language differences and varying communication styles, can further complicate teamwork, making active listening and adaptability essential for effective collaboration. Addressing these challenges requires a comprehensive understanding of cultural contexts, alongside the development of inclusive practices that value all voices within the therapeutic process, ultimately enhancing the effectiveness of music therapy in promoting well-being for diverse clients.

References

Archard, D., & Skivenes, M. (2009). Balancing a child's best interests and the child's views. *International Journal of Children's Rights, 17*(1), 1–21.

Baines, S. (2013). Music therapy as an anti-oppressive practice. *The Arts in Psychotherapy, 40*(1), 1–5. https://doi.org/10.1016/j.aip.2012.09.003

Beckmann, H. B. (2013). Music, adolescents and health: Narratives about how young people use music as a health resource in daily life. In *Musical life stories: Narratives on health musicking* (Vol. 6). Centre for Music and Health Publication Series, NMH-publikasjoner

Bell, S. A. (2016). *A music therapist's self-reflection on her aboriginal heritage: A heuristic self-inquiry* (Master's thesis). Concordia University, Montreal.

Bolger, L. (2013). Music therapy and international development in action and reflection: A case study of a women's music group in rural Bangladesh. *Australian Journal of Music Therapy, 23*, 22–38.

Brodie, E., Cowling, E., Nissen, N., Paine, A., Jochum, V., & Warburton, D. (2009). *Understanding participation: A literature review*. NCVO.

Brown, J. M. (2002). Towards a culturally centered music therapy practice. *Voices: A World Forum for Music Therapy, 2*(1). https://doi.org/10.15845/voices.v2i1.72

Bruscia, K. E. (1998). *The dynamics of music psychotherapy*. Barcelona Publishers.

Bruscia, K. E. (2015). *Reflexivity in music therapy: An anthology*. Barcelona Publishers.

Caló, F., Steiner, A., Millar, S., & Teasdale, S. (2020). The impact of a community-based music intervention on the health and well-being of young people: A realist evaluation. *Health & Social Care in the Community, 28*(3), 988–997.

Chase, K. M. (2004). Therapy with gay and lesbian clients: Implications for music therapists. *Music Therapy Perspectives, 22*(1), 34–38. https://doi.org/10.1093/mtp/22.1.34

Cobbett, S. (2016). Context and relationships: Using the systemic approach with music therapy in work with children, adolescents, and their families. *British Journal of Music Therapy, 30*(2), 65–73.

Costa-Giomi, E. (2004). Effects of three years of piano instruction on children's academic achievement, school performance, and self-esteem. *Psychology of Music, 32*(2), 139–152. https://doi.org/10.1177/0305735604032002004

Cotter, K. E., & Krüger, V. (in press). Music therapy and family systems theory. In M. Viega, A. dos Santos, & B. Wheeler (Eds.), *Music therapy handbook*. Guildford Press.

DeBacker, J. (1993). Containment in music therapy. In M. H. Heal & T. Wigram (Eds.), *Music therapy in health and education* (pp. 93–39). Jessica Kingsley Publisher.

DeNora, T. (2007). Health and music in everyday life: A theory of practice. *Psyke & Logos, 28*, 271–287.

Derrington, P. (2019). "What's the WiFi code here?": Connecting with adolescents in music therapy. In K. McFerran, P. Derrington, & S. Saarikallio (Eds.), *Handbook of music, adolescents, and well-being* (pp. 165–175). Oxford University Press.

Donley, J. (2020). Multicultural experiential learning in music therapy supervision. *Voices: A World Forum for Music Therapy, 20*(1), 1–2020. https://doi.org/10.15845/voices.v20i1.3005

Fairchild, R., & McFerran, K. S. (2019). "Music is everything": Using collaborative group songwriting as an arts-based method with children experiencing homelessness and family violence. *Nordic Journal of Music Therapy, 28*(2), 88–107. https://doi.org/10.1080/08098131.2018.1530189

Fairchild, R., & Sheridan, J. (2018). Strengthening bonds between children, young people, and their families after family violence. *Voices: A World Forum for Music Therapy, 18*(4), 1–13. https://doi.org/10.15845/voices.v18i4.2600

Fairchild, R., Thompson, G., & McFerran, K. S. (2017). Exploring the meaning of a performance in music therapy for children and their families experiencing homelessness and family violence. *Music Therapy Perspectives, 35*(1), 36–49. https://doi.org/10.1093/mtp/miw004

Gill, A., & Rickard, N. S. (2012). Non-musical benefits of school-based music education and training. In N. S. Rickard & K. McFerran (Eds.), *Lifelong engagement with music: Benefits for mental health and well-being* (pp. 57–72). Nova. https://doi.org/10.15845/voices.v23i1.3642

Gold, C., Saarikallio, S., Crooke, A. H. D., & McFerran, K. S. (2017). Group music therapy as a preventive intervention for young people at risk: A cluster-randomized trial. *Journal of Music Therapy, 54*(2), 133–160.

Gonzalez, P. J. (2011). The impact of music therapists' music cultures on the development of their professional frameworks. *Qualitative Inquiries in Music Therapy, 6*, 1–33.

Gouk, P. (2017). Introduction. In P. Gouk (Ed.), *Musical healing in cultural contexts* (pp. 1–25). Routledge.

Hadley, S., & Norris, M. S. (2016). Musical multicultural competency in music therapy: The first step. *Music Therapy Perspectives, 34*(2), 129–137.

Haering, S. I. (2022). *The impact of music therapy on children in a multicultural elementary school* (1st ed.). Springer Fachmedien Wiesbaden. https://doi.org/10.1007/978-3-658-39330-4

Hussey, D. L., Reed, A. M., Laymann, D. L., & Pasiali, V. (2007). Music therapy and complex trauma: A protocol for developing social reciprocity. *Residential Treatment for Children & Youth, 24*(1–2), 111–129. https://doi.org/10.1300/J007v24n01_07

Jacobsen, S. L. (2019). Musikterapi i udredning og behandling af udsatte børn og familier. *Tidsskriftet Norges Barnevern, 96*(1–2), 56–68.

Johns, U. (2017). Når musikk skaper nye bevegelsesmuligheter for traumatiserte barn [When music creates new movement possibilities for traumatized children]. In K. Stensæth, G. Trondalen, & Ø. Varkøy (Eds.), *Musikk, handlinger, muligheter: Festskrift til Even Ruud [Even Ruud, Music Therapy in Child Welfare Memorial Volume]* (pp. 107–123). Centre for Music and Health, CREAMAH.

Jones, P., Cedar, L., Coleman, A., Haythorne, D., Mercieca, D., & Ramsden, E. (2021). *Child agency and voice in therapy: New ways of working in the arts therapies*. Routledge.

Klyve, G. P., & Rolvsjord, R. (2022). Moments of fun: Narratives of children's experiences of music therapy in mental health care. *Nordic Journal of Music Therapy, 32*(2), 100–120. https://doi.org/10.1080/08098131.2022.2055114

Knijn, T., & van Nijnatten, C. (2011). Child welfare in The Netherlands: Between privacy and protection. In N. Gilbert, N. Parton, & M. Skivenes (Eds.), *Child protection systems: International trends and orientations* (Online ed.). Oxford Academic. https://doi.org/10.1093/acprof:oso/9780199793358.003.0011

van der Kolk, B. (2014). *The body keeps the score: Brain, mind, and body in the healing of trauma*. Viking.

Krüger, V. (2016). Musikk som ressurs for ungdommers livslange læringsbehov—Et tverrfaglig eksempel fra skolen og barnevernets praksis [Music as a resource for adolescents' life-long learning processes: An interdisciplinary case example from school and child welfare]. In L. Stensæth, V. Krüger, & S. Fuglestad (Eds.), *I transitt mellom til og fra: Tekster om musikk og deltakelse i barnevern [In transit—Between toward and from: Texts about music and participation in a child welfare setting]*. Norwegian Academy of Music.

Krüger, V. (2020). *Music therapy in child welfare: Bridging provision, protection, and participation*. Barcelona Publishers.

Krüger, V., & Tuastad, L. (2025). The Lil Peep paradox—The role of professional discretion when dealing with complex idioms from popular culture. *iNordic Journal of Music Therapy*, 1–16. https://doi.org/10.1080/08098131.2025.2465758

Krüger, V., Risnes, T., Nilsen, C. S., & Høiseth, T. (2019). Musikkterapi og skoledeltakelse for ungdommer med barnevernsbakgrunn—en casestudie [Music therapy and school participation for youth with a child welfare background—A case study]. *Norges Barnevern, 96*(1–2), 40–55.

Krüger, V., Crooke, A., Solberg, D., & Sæle, E. (2023). Exploring the potential for music therapy to support 21st century education goals: Interviews with six Norwegian teachers. *Voices: A World Forum for Music Therapy, 23*(1). https://doi.org/10.15845/voices.v23i1.3642

Langford, M., Skivenes, M., Søvig, K. H., & Loven Kirkebø, T. (2019). Introduction: Implementing child rights. In M. Langford, M. Skivenes, & K. H. Søvig (Eds.), *Children's rights in Norway: An implementation paradox?* (pp. 15–41). Universitetsforlaget.

Lansdown, G. (2011). *Every child's right to be heard: A resource guide on the UN Committee on the Rights of the Child General Comment No.12.* Save the Children/UNICEF.

Lundy, L. (2007). 'Voice' is not enough: Conceptualising Article 12 of the United Nations Convention on the Rights of the Child. *British Educational Research Journal, 33*(6), 927–942.

Lundy, L., McEvoy, L., & Byrne, B. (2011). Working with young children as co-researchers: An approach informed by the United Nations Convention on the Rights of the Child. *Early Education and Development, 22*(5), 714–736.

MacDonald, R., Kreutz, G., & Mitchell, L. (Eds.). (2013). *Music, health, and wellbeing.* Oxford University Press.

Mahoney, E. R. (2015). *Multicultural music therapy: An exploration* [Position paper]. *Voices: A World Forum for Music Therapy, 15*(2). https://doi.org/10.15845/voices.v15i2.832

McFerran, K. S., & Teggelove, T. (2011). Music therapy with young people in schools: After the Black Saturday fires. *Voices: A World Forum for Music Therapy, 11*(1).

Miell, D. E., MacDonald, R. A. R., & Hargreaves, D. J. (2005). *Musical communication.* Oxford University Press.

Nöcker-Ribaupierre, M., & Wölfl, A. (2010). Music to counter violence: A preventative approach for working with adolescents in schools. *Nordic Journal of Music Therapy, 19*(2), 151–161. https://doi.org/10.1080/08098131.2010.489997

Pavlicevic, M. (2003). *Groups in music: Strategies from music therapy.* Jessica Kingsley Publishers.

Rickson, D., & McFerran, K. (2014). *Creating music cultures in the schools: A perspective from community music therapy.* Barcelona Publishers.

Rolvsjord, R. (2010). *Resource-oriented music therapy in mental health care.* Barcelona Publishers.

Ruud, E. (1998). *Music therapy, improvisation, communication, and culture.* Barcelona Publishers.

Ruud, E. (2010). *Music therapy: A perspective from the humanities.* Barcelona Publishers.

Saarikallio, S. (2019). Music as a resource for agency and empowerment in identity construction. In K. McFerran, P. Derrington, & S. Saarikallio (Eds.), *Handbook of music, adolescents, and well-being* (pp. 89–99). Oxford University Press.

dos Santos, A. (2024). Nurturing our reflexivity. *Nordic Journal of Music Therapy, 33*(1), 1–3. https://doi.org/10.1080/08098131.2023.2282814

Scrine, E. (2019). Reframing intervention and inclusion: The importance of exploring gender and sexuality in music therapy with all young people. In *Handbook of music, adolescents, and wellbeing* (pp. 151–161). Oxford University Press.

Siegel, D. J. (2012). *The developing mind: How relationships and the brain interact to shape who we are* (3rd ed.). Guilford Press.

Stige, B. (2002). *Culture-centered music therapy*. Barcelona Publishers.

Sutton, J. (2002). Trauma in context. In J. Sutton (Ed.), *Music, music therapy, and trauma: International perspectives* (pp. 21–41). Jessica Kingsley Publishers.

Teachout, D. J. (2005). The impact of music education on a child's growth and development. Sounds of learning. *International Foundation for Music Research, 46*(4), 568–587.

Trondalen, G. (2016). *Relational music therapy: An intersubjective perspective*. Barcelona Publishers.

Uhlig, S., Jansen, E., & Scherder, E. (2018). "Being a bully isn't very cool...": Rap & sing music therapy for enhanced emotional self-regulation in an adolescent school setting - a randomized controlled trial. *Psychology of Music, 46*(4), 568–587. https://doi.org/10.1177/0305735617719154

UNCHR. (2008). *Guidelines on determining the best interests of the child*. https://www.unhcr.org

Zanders, M. L. (2015). Music therapy practices and processes with foster-care youth: Formulating an approach to clinical work. *Music Therapy Perspectives, 33*(2), 97–107.

CHAPTER 3

Integrating Sociocultural Perspectives into Music Therapy: Advancing the Best Interests of the Child

Introduction

This chapter focuses on perspectives from music therapy to situate the best interest of the child within the sociocultural factors influencing a child's life. Additionally, the perspectives outlined in this chapter have been utilized in texts about music therapy and children, rendering them representative of the various discourses in the field. As discussed in the previous chapter, the term "children" necessitates a sociocultural understanding that provides us with a contextual view of how cultural differences must be taken into consideration when making decisions about a child's well-being or health.

Sociocultural perspectives on childhood contrast with the traditional view of childhood as a static and universal concept. Moreover, critical perspectives are needed to balance the elements described in the best interest of the child (see previous chapter). Understanding the ecology of children's development is essential, but there is also a need for a critical perspective on child development and childhood. We will also highlight the current development in the music therapy literature related to critical thinking and evaluation of traditional music therapy approaches. These perspectives include post-humanism and disability. Advocates for these perspectives view childhood as socially constructed, shaped by the specific

"It was fun." ("Fredrik," in Klyve and Rolvsjord, 2023, p. 109)

V. Krüger, K. M. Murphy, *Child-Centred Music Therapy*,
https://doi.org/10.1007/978-3-031-85724-9_3

societies and cultures of different times and places. Sociocultural factors influence norms and values regarding child-rearing, education, and family structures. It is important to remember that what is considered in the best interest of a child in one culture may not be the same in another.

Resource-Oriented Music Therapy

Resource-Oriented Music Therapy (ROMT) is an approach to music therapy practice that focuses on identifying and utilizing the strengths, abilities, and resources of individuals and groups to promote well-being and facilitate growth and healing (Rolvsjord, 2010). In ROMT, the therapist collaborates with clients to identify their existing resources, such as musical skills, personal strengths, social support networks, cultural practices, and resilience factors. The therapist then works with the clients using these resources to address their therapeutic goals and needs. This approach, while developed in her work with adults, can easily be applied to music therapy with children. ROMT provides the theoretical grounding for recent studies in which participation in music therapy by children and adolescents was investigated (Klyve & Rolvsjord, 2022). Referring to Article 31 in the UNCRC (1989), Klyve (2019) highlights children's right to engage in play. Play is often regarded as the child's language by most child development theorists most prominent among them being Stern et al. and Malloch and Trevarthen (2009). Music therapists can support children's play, helping them to regulate and express emotions. Additionally, they are trained to engage in children's play, attuning to their expressions, using other modalities than words, such as sound and gestures, to build relationships. Furthermore, musical play fosters creativity and imagination, essential components of cognitive and emotional development. Additionally, play serves as a vehicle for social interaction, enabling children to develop essential social skills, build relationships, and foster a sense of belonging (Winnicott, 2005). The following principles of resource-oriented music therapy can be used in work with children (Klyve et al., 2023).

Strength-Based Approach: ROMT emphasizes identifying and building upon the strengths and assets rather than focusing solely on deficits or problems. By highlighting existing resources, children can be empowered to take an active role in their therapeutic process and work towards positive outcomes.

(*continued*)

(continued)
Child-Centred approach: ROMT is inherently child-centred, with the therapist respecting and valuing the unique perspectives, preferences, and experiences of each individual child. Therapy goals and interventions are tailored to meet the specific needs and preferences of the child.

Collaborative Process: ROMT involves a collaborative partnership between the therapist and the child, with both parties working together towards shared goals.

Holistic Approach: ROMT considers the whole person, addressing physical, emotional, cognitive, social, and spiritual aspects of well-being. Music is used as a holistic tool to engage clients on multiple levels and promote integrated healing.

Culturally Responsive Practice: ROMT acknowledges and respects the cultural backgrounds, values, and beliefs of clients, incorporating culturally relevant music and practices into therapy sessions as appropriate. Cultural resources are recognized as valuable assets in promoting well-being (Inspired by Rolvsjord, 2010 and Klyve & Rolvsjord, 2022).

Culture-Centred Music Therapy

Stige (2002) posits that cultural experiences can promote socialization which can improve the person's quality of life, and they note that music therapists should consider culture in their clinical work. According to Stige, music therapy is not "culture free," but influenced by the norms, values, and beliefs of both the client and the therapist. Stige further encourages music therapists to adjust their approach to music therapy clinical work based on the client's beliefs about music, health, and therapy. Stige is, among others, inspired by the work of Vygotsky (1978), who famously examined the relationship between culture, context, and learning. Vygotsky's sociocultural theory highlights the role of social and cultural factors in cognitive development. It emphasizes the importance of social interactions, language, and cultural contexts in shaping a child's learning and development. Sociocultural theories of development offer an alternative understanding of child development adding a new framework in which to consider children's rights. Vygotsky (1978) saw development as a process arising out of participation in the social and intellectual life surrounding the child. While Vygotsky did not specifically focus on music in his theory, his ideas can be applied to understanding how music fits into the sociocultural context of human development and learning.

Vygotsky's sociocultural theory provides a framework for understanding how music is learned, understood, and integrated into one's identity within a cultural and social context. It emphasizes the importance of social interactions, cultural tools, and guidance from more knowledgeable individuals in the process of musical development and learning. What is often referred to as the second generation of sociocultural theorists (Lave & Wenger, 1991) is also relevant in the context of music therapy for children and adolescents. Their theory highlights the importance of social and cultural contexts in the learning process. Their theory has been used in numerous studies in music therapy (e.g. Enge & Stige, 2022; Krüger, 2019). Lave and Wenger suggest that learning occurs within "communities of practice," where individuals engage in shared activities and develop a shared identity. In music therapy–related activities, children often participate in musical communities of practice, such as school bands, choirs, or music classes. These communities provide a context for children to learn from each other and from more experienced musicians, like older peers. Lave and Wenger propose the term "legitimate peripheral participation," meaning that newcomers to a community of practice start as peripheral participants and gradually move towards more central roles as they gain expertise. In a music therapy context, participants often start with simple musical activities and gradually become more involved in complex music-making as they gain proficiency. For instance, a child may begin by playing basic melodies on an instrument and later become a part of a larger ensemble. Participation in a musical community of practice contributes to the development of an individual's identity and meaning. In the realm of music therapy, children's involvement in musical communities helps shape their musical identity and the meaning they attach to music. Through shared experiences and interactions, children develop a deeper understanding of the cultural and emotional significance of music.

Community Music Therapy

Community music therapy is grounded by the central values found in the Universal Declaration of Human Rights including freedom, equality, respect, and solidarity (Stige & Aarø, 2012, p. 196). Music creates possibilities for action and for forming community from the perspective of CoMT (Stige & Aarø, 2012, p. 15). Possibilities for growth and creation of community occur as we interact with others through music. Music therapists and individuals bring knowledge and experience to the space and together they engage in meaningful musical interactions. The therapist's focus is not on fixing an issue, but on providing a space where people bring their culture and way of being. The qualities of community music therapy practice, informed by research, were synthesized in the acronym PREPARE which stands for participatory, resource oriented, ecological, performative, activistic, reflective, and ethic driven (Stige & Aarø, 2012, pp. 18–20).

The participatory quality of CoMT refers to the intentional opportunities for individual and social participation within the therapeutic process. This is characterized by collaborative and democratic relationships with a focus on human rights, mutual empowerment, and collaborative decision-making.

The resource-oriented quality reflects that the focus is on the mobilization of personal, social, cultural, and material resources within the community where the therapeutic process is undertaken. This approach focuses on both the development and access of resources to improve health and wellness.

The ecological quality of CoMT reflects the importance of the various aspects of environment to personal and communal health. Therefore, the therapeutic focus is not limited to individuals, and includes the reciprocal relationships between individuals, groups, and networks.

The performative quality refers to work with human and social development through action. This involves use of the performative possibilities of music as action, and it might or might not include performances understood as gigs or concerts in a social context. Explorations of opportunities for expression and development of self and social systems are central.

(*continued*)

(continued)

The activist quality acknowledges that health and wellness as communal issues and the core issues of participants are linked to human rights issues and limitations in society. This may require the community music therapist to take on roles and responsibilities outside the traditional definition of a therapist.

The reflective quality is an expansion of the participatory quality to include all stakeholders in the understanding and processing the outcomes of the therapeutic process. This impacts the practice and research process of CoMT.

The ethics driven quality of CoMT reflexts that human rights are? the organizing principle of this approach. Values of freedom, mutual respect, equality, and solidarity are central to the therapeutic process (Inspired by Stige & Aarø, 2012, pp. 15–17).

Being part of a community enables the citizen to access resources, interacting with others, experience mutuality, shared expression, and interconnectedness. Epp (2007) acknowledges that traditional music therapy literature romanticizes music as a direct representation of self and she argues that music therapists "cannot detach expressive content from the live performance of music" (Epp, 2007, p. 1). This view fits well with sociocultural theorists such as Bronfenbrenner's (1979) ecological systems theory which emphasizes the influence of multiple environmental systems (microsystem, mesosystem, exosystem, macrosystem, and chronosystem) on a child's development. Ecological system theory focuses on the interconnectedness of various contexts and how they shape a child's experiences. As noted by Bronfenbrenner (1979), a child's opportunity to master life is connected to sociocultural factors such as attachment to peers and adults, reciprocity in relationships, progressive complexity in learning activities, and balance of power (Bronfenbrenner, 1979, p. 46).

Microsystem: The micro system is the most immediate and direct environment that directly influences a child. It includes the child's family, school, peers, and community. To determine the best interest of the child, it's crucial to consider the quality of interactions and relationships within these microsystems. In terms of a sociocultural view on music, this level would involve how family members or close friends influence a child's musical exposure and participation.

Mesosystem: The mesosystem involves the connections and interactions between different microsystems. For example, how a child's family interacts with their school can significantly impact the child's development. Regarding music, this might involve how a child's school experiences, and family life intersect to influence their musical interests and opportunities.

Exosystem: The exosystem includes external settings or institutions that indirectly influence the child. For instance, a parent's workplace policies can affect the family environment and, in turn, the child's well-being. In terms of music, this level might involve the availability of music therapy, community music programmes, or the presence of local music organizations.

Macrosystem: The macrosystem encompasses the broader cultural, societal, and ideological context in which the child lives. Cultural norms, values, and social policies can profoundly affect the child's development. In the context of music, this level might influence the types of music that are promoted or valued within a culture.

Chronosystem: The chronosystem recognizes that development is a dynamic process over time. Life events, historical events, and the timing of experiences all play a role in determining what is in the best interest of the child at a particular point in time. This could include the impact of significant life events on a child's relationship with music, such as moving to a new place with different musical traditions or experiencing a family crisis that affects their access to music education (Inspired by Bronfenbrenner, 1979).

Trauma and Resilience-Informed Music Therapy

The increased awareness of the impact of trauma on childhood development has led to an increase in the use of trauma-informed care (TIC) framework in work with children (Bath, 2015). TIC emphasizes creating safe and supportive environments for children who have experienced trauma. This framework helps therapists recognize the profound and multifaceted impact of trauma on individuals' physical, emotional, and mental health, aiming to minimize further harm (Substance Abuse and Mental Health Services Administration [SAMHSA], 2014). A trauma-informed approach to working with children seeks to create environments where children feel safe, valued, and capable of building trusting relationships, which are essential for healing.

Neuroscientific research has demonstrated that music can play a vital role in work with children who have experienced trauma by decreasing physiological arousal and modulating activity in brain structures involved in emotional and motivational processes (Koelsch, 2015). For instance, studies have shown that engaging with music can lower levels of the stress hormone cortisol, facilitating relaxation and emotional regulation. This is particularly important for children who have faced trauma, as they often experience heightened states of arousal that can impede their ability to engage socially and learn effectively.

Moreover, advances in neuroscience have led to a better understanding of brain development in children, with research indicating that music profoundly influences various aspects of cognitive, emotional, and social development (Toader et al., 2023). For example, musical training has been linked to improved language skills, enhanced memory, and greater emotional intelligence. Music serves as a universal phenomenon that transcends barriers, providing a means for children to express themselves and connect with others, fostering social skills and emotional resilience.

This perspective is further supported by Siegel (2012), who suggests that emotional stimulation is crucial for the proper development of the brain. Siegel emphasizes the importance of positive interactions and emotional experiences in shaping the neural pathways that underlie cognitive and emotional functioning. By integrating music into therapeutic and educational practices, practitioners can leverage its ability to stimulate emotional and social development, helping children build connections and navigate their experiences more effectively.

Trauma-informed care has gained significant attention as it provides a less intrusive way of addressing the long-term effects of adverse childhood experiences (ACEs) on physical and mental health outcomes. ACEs, which include experiences such as abuse, neglect, and household dysfunction, have been strongly linked to the development of chronic medical conditions, psychiatric disorders, and maladaptive behaviours in adulthood. Felitti and Anda (2010) note that early exposure to trauma can disrupt neurodevelopment, leading to increased vulnerability to both physical and psychological illnesses later in life. Their research highlights the importance of integrating trauma-informed approaches in healthcare settings to mitigate these negative outcomes. By recognizing the profound and lasting impact of ACEs, trauma-informed care emphasizes safety, trust, and empowerment, aiming to create supportive environments where individuals can heal, and the risk of re-traumatization is reduced.

Abrahams et al. (2024) conducted a scoping review of 35 peer-reviewed articles published between 2000 and 2022 and identified 173 music therapy interventions addressing 20 ACEs and 83 treatment goals. They found only four studies demonstrated significant effects on varying outcomes. The review highlights the diversity in interventions and goals but notes that inconsistent reporting hampers the ability to draw firm conclusions. The authors recommend standardized documentation of music therapy practices to enhance clarity and comparability.

Despite lack of evidence in terms of standardized documentation, a wide variety of literature demonstrate that music therapists are increasingly working with trauma survivors engaging them in music-based experiences (e.g. Heiderscheit & Murphy, 2021; Sokira et al., 2023). Safety built through music therapy can lead to the development of trusting relationships for trauma survivors (Perryman et al., 2019). A sense of safety is created when the participants' feelings are understood by the therapist (dos Santos, 2018), the therapists are authentic in their interactions with participants (Perryman et al., 2019) and provide a safe and supportive environment (Hussey et al., 2007). Strehlow (2009) and Christenbury (2017) demonstrated that giving some form of control to the individual over the session may help them to establish their own form of security. Engaging in music-making activities encourages individuals to share experiences, express emotions, and work together towards common goals, which can strengthen their connections. This process not only promotes the development of interpersonal skills but also positions individuals to take on leadership or co-leadership roles within the group.

The literature highlights the critical role peers play in providing social support, emphasizing that positive peer interactions contribute to emotional well-being and resilience (Enge & Stige, 2022). Connection between group members may establish a sense of safety through sharing and discussing music activities. Research findings note that participants in music therapy groups felt safe enough to express their feelings in songs when they felt they were supported by the therapist in the songwriting process (Viega, 2016; Zanders, 2015). Resilience theory (Sokira et al., 2023) explores how children can overcome adversity and thrive despite challenging circumstances. Resilience theory focuses on identifying protective factors and strategies that promote resilience in children. Adults and peers play an important role in how children build resilience, and research shows that children who have strong relationships with caring adults who believe in them are more likely to be resilient (Masten & Tellegen, 2012). These relationships provide children with a sense of security and belonging, helping them to cope with stress and adversity. Moreover, children who have a strong social support network are more likely to be resilient. This network can provide them with emotional support, practical help, and a sense of belonging.

Critical Childhood Studies and Music Therapy

Equity and Access: Considering critical childhood studies, music therapy has the potential to address disparities in healthcare access by providing services to underserved populations, including those with limited financial resources, physical disabilities, mental health challenges, or marginalized identities.

Cultural Humility Music therapists strive to develop culturally competent practices that honour the unique cultural perspectives, traditions, and values of their clients. By integrating culturally relevant music, rituals, and traditions into therapy sessions, music therapists can create a safe and inclusive space for clients to explore their identities and address social and systemic barriers to well-being.

(*continued*)

(continued)

Advocacy and Activism: Music therapists often engage in advocacy and activism to promote social justice and systemic change within their profession and communities. This may involve advocating for policies that increase access to music therapy services, collaborating with community organizations to address social determinants of health.

Empowerment and Social Change: Music therapy interventions can empower individuals and communities to voice their experiences, advocate for their needs, and effect social change. Through songwriting, improvisation, and performance, clients can express their stories, raise awareness about social issues, and mobilize support for collective action.

Community Building and Solidarity: Music therapy promotes community building and solidarity by bringing people together in shared musical experiences. By creating spaces where individuals can share their stories, validate each other's experiences, and work towards common goals, music therapy strengthens social bonds and promotes social justice values such as equity, diversity, and solidarity.

Childhood as Evolving: Music therapy encompasses a view of childhood where children actively shape their identities through technology, with children's rights being relational, emphasizing connection and participation rather than just protection.

The previous section presented perspectives that are relevant to understand the relationships and practices in music therapy that involve children. Houston (2017) suggests professionals working with children and adolescents should also cast a critical, reflexive gaze over their own profession. Therefore, music therapists not only need to understand the ecology of children's development, but there is also a need for a critical perspective of the same. In this section we will give a brief overview of critical childhood studies (CCS) which brings together academic fields and theoretical orientations. CCS concerns research with children, youth, families, and communities in diverse social contexts, and seeks to explore, understand, and theorize diverse childhoods and what it means to be a young person in the world today. Usually, CCS researchers use qualitative, ethnographic, and participatory methodologies to develop insights into the lifeworld of differently gendered, abled, classed, raced, positioned, and cultured children and youths. These approaches to knowledge production are usually critical and reflexive. Critical childhood studies focus on how children's actions can influence, challenge and contest the established ordering of society, or structure an ideology. Historical academic figures such as Marx (1867/1990), Weber (1978), Arendt (1951), and Durkheim (1951) can be seen as important figures, giving direction to how we understand society in terms of its structures, boundaries, institutions, establishments, and wider social relations. Marx's (1867/1990) ideas on social inequality and class dynamics shed light on how socioeconomic factors shape children's access to therapeutic resources. Weber's (1978) concepts of authority and bureaucracy help analyse the institutional structures governing child welfare systems, impacting how services like music therapy are administered. Arendt's (1951) focus on the impact of oppressive systems on personal freedom can be applied to understanding how societal structures may limit or empower children. Music therapy, as a tool for emotional expression and self-discovery, aligns with Arendt's belief in the importance of autonomy and resistance to oppressive forces. Durkheim's (1951) focus on social integration and the role of collective norms may inform the importance of fostering social bonds and emotional resilience in children through music therapy.

Giddens' (1990) theory of structuration, which emphasizes the interplay between individual agency and social structures, offers a dynamic framework to explore how children and therapists co-construct healing spaces, ensuring their voices and interests are central to therapeutic processes. Giddens (1984) argues that agency is always related to structure—hence his agency/structure framework relates to the notion of power. Agency is thus the capacity of social actors to act—to impact a change that has positive effects for themselves, those around them, the society, and the planet. This idea of agency is relevant both to children and to adults alike, and allows the transformative power of these actors, and their influence on their lives, or on the conditions of any structure of societal, or minority groups. The concern of how much "real" agency and capacity children must have to effect change—given the conditions of surrounding structures, the reproduction of society, ideology, culture, ethnicity, and politics involved in each situation—is one of the challenges that childhood studies work with, research, and think about (Wyness, 2012).

The published literature in music therapy began to have a critical focus in the beginning of the twenty-first century. These studies, many of them theoretical explorations and positions papers, usually challenge structures in society as they explore the relationship outside the narrow therapist-client encounter, looking at relationships between societies, individuals, music, and health (e.g. Ansdell, 2002). Critical childhood studies examine childhood as a social and cultural construct and challenge traditional notions of childhood. This research has important implications for how we understand and treat children, and for how we create societies that are more supportive of their well-being. Comte's (2016) exploration of the underlying neo-colonial dynamics present in music therapy practices with refugee populations is relevant for this discussion. She critically examines how music therapists' approaches may unintentionally perpetuate power imbalances rooted in colonial histories highlighting the need for music therapists to become more aware of cultural sensitivities, and to adopt practices that are less about imposing Western ideals and more about engaging in culturally responsive and collaborative approaches. The paper calls for reflection on ethical practices, urging professionals to reassess their roles to avoid reinforcing existing inequities in therapeutic settings.

Post-humanistic Perspectives on Music Therapy and Children

Post-humanism is another perspective relevant for CSS. A post-humanistic perspective in music therapy challenges the traditional human-centred approaches by emphasizing relationality, interconnectedness, and the importance of non-human elements in therapeutic contexts. When applied to children's rights, this perspective broadens the understanding of agency and participation, viewing children not as passive recipients of care but as active participants whose interactions with their environment, technology, and music are integral to their well-being. Fortin (2006) argues that children's rights must be adapted to modern societal shifts, which resonates with post-humanism's call for recognizing the dynamic, non-linear nature of children's engagement. This inclusive perspective enriches the discourse on how children's rights are enacted and respected, ensuring a more holistic approach to their emotional, social, and developmental needs.

Post-human theories suggest that childhood, like other aspects of human existence, is undergoing a transformation in the context of emerging technologies, ecological concerns, and evolving understandings of identity and agency. These theories acknowledge that children's experiences and identities are increasingly shaped by digital technologies, artificial intelligence, and other non-human elements (Murris, 2016). Post-humanist perspectives suggest that children are not simply passive recipients of technological influences but are active participants in shaping their identities through interactions with technology. Post-humanism scholars argue that children's rights should be understood as relational rights, that is, rights that are defined in relation to other people, technologies, and things (Malone et al., 2020). This means that children's rights are not just about protecting them from harm, but also about enabling children to connect with others and to participate in their communities, for example, through digital technologies (UNICEF Office of Research—Innocenti, n.d.). As such, post-humanistic thought challenges conventional notions of what it means to be a child and how children relate to the world.

In music therapy literature, post-human theory follows a line of thinking that can be traced back to scholars such as Kenny (2006), Rolvsjord (2010), and Hadley (2006). Common for these scholars is a belief that music therapy should challenge traditional notions of what it means to be human and how humans relate to the world, including the concept of childhood. Metell (2019) takes ideas from queer theories and disability studies arguing that there is a need to reflect on how we talk and write about music therapy practices with disabled children as well as to challenge the concepts and attitudes towards diversity to contribute to inclusive environments that appreciates and celebrates diversity. Queer theories and disability studies challenge the idea that there is a single standard of "normal" or "healthy" and argue that all bodies and minds are valuable. Shaw (2022) developed Post-Ableist Music Therapy (PAMT) using post-humanism as a foundation. She explains PAMT as a creative process that seeks to work with a person and community to provide an environment and experience that is less disabling through addressing ableist barriers, exploring connections, and providing new and less restrictive spaces through primarily musical or music-related experiences. It welcomes different ways of being and resists a one-size-fits-all approach. Instead, the process is guided by the people involved and their contexts guide the process. Shaw builds on Foucault's (1982) ideas about agonism. Agonism understands the struggle between ethical standpoints as a potential site of productive possibility (agonistic struggle). Following this line of reasoning, Scrine

(2021) describes the ways in which music therapy can respond to power relations as they occur within and beyond "trauma-informed" spaces. She highlights two overarching potentials for music therapy within a shifting trauma paradigm: (1) as a site in which to reframe perceived risk by fostering young people's resistance and building their political agency and (2) in challenging the assumption of "safe spaces" and instead moving towards practices of "structuring safety."

In structuring safety, practitioners continuously navigate consent, create opportunities for clients to exercise choice and control, and remain curious about their acts of resistance in the face of oppression. Music therapy offers powerful potential here as individuals move from subject or object and into an active participant. At music therapists' disposal lies not only the elements of music that afford structure, predictability, and flexibility, but also infinite opportunities to offer choice and control, which are crucial in cultivating a culture of consent between therapist and client (Scrine, 2021, p. 12).

References

Abrahams, T., van de Ree, M., Hakvoort, L., Konijn, C., Otten, R., Popma, A., & Nijhof, K. (2024). Music therapy and adverse childhood experiences: A scoping review. *Nordic Journal of Music Therapy*. https://doi.org/10.1080/08098131.2024.2388885

Ansdell, G. (2002). Community music therapy & the winds of change. *Voices: A World Forum for Music Therapy, 2*(2), 1–46. https://doi.org/10.15845/voices.v2i2.83

Arendt, H. (1951). *The origins of totalitarianism*. Harcourt Brace.

Bath, H. (2015). The three pillars of trauma-wise care: Healing in the other 23 hours. *Reclaiming Children and Youth, 23*(4), 44–46.

Bronfenbrenner, U. (1979). *The ecology of human development: Experiments by nature and design*. Harvard University Press.

Christenbury, K. R. (2017). I will follow you: The combined use of songwriting and art to promote healing in a child who has been traumatized. *Music Therapy Perspectives, 35*(1), 1–12. https://doi.org/10.1093/mtp/miv005

Comte, R. (2016). Neo-colonialism in music therapy: A critical interpretive synthesis of the literature concerning music therapy practice with refugees. *Voices: A World Forum for Music Therapy, 16*(3). https://doi.org/10.15845/voices.v16i3.865

Durkheim, È. (1951). *Suicide: A study in sociology* (J. A. Spaulding & G. Simpson, Trans.). The Free Press. (Original work published 1897).

Enge, K. E. A., & Stige, B. (2022). Musical pathways to the peer community: A collective case study of refugee children's use of music therapy. *Nordic Journal of Music Therapy, 31*(1), 7–24. https://doi.org/10.1080/08098131.2021.1891130

Epp, E. (2007). Locating the autonomous voice: Self-expression in music-centered music therapy. *Voices: A World Forum for Music Therapy, 7*(1). https://doi.org/10.15845/voices.v7i1.463

Felitti, V. J., & Anda, R. F. (2010). The relationship of adverse childhood experiences to adult medical disease, psychiatric disorders, and sexual behavior: Implications for healthcare. In R. Lanius & E. Vermette (Eds.), *The hidden epidemic: The impact of early life trauma on health and disease* (pp. 77–87). Cambridge University Press.

Fortin, J. (2006). Accommodating children's rights in a post-human rights act era. *The Modern Law Review, 69*(3), 299–326. https://www.jstor.org/stable/3699029

Foucault, M. (1982). The subject and power. *Critical Inquiry, 8*(4), 777–795. https://doi.org/10.1086/448181

Giddens, A. (1984). *The constitution of society: Outline of the theory of structuration.* University of California Press.

Giddens, A. (1990). *The consequences of modernity.* Polity Press.

Hadley, S. (Ed.). (2006). *Feminist perspectives in music therapy.* Barcelona Publishers.

Heiderscheit, A., & Murphy, K. M. (2021). Trauma-informed care in music therapy: Principles, guidelines, and a clinical case illustration. *Music Therapy Perspectives, 39*(2), 142–151.

Houston, S. (2017). Towards a critical ecology of child development in social work: Aligning the theories of Bronfenbrenner and Bourdieu. *Families, Relationships and Societies, 6*(1), 53–69. https://doi.org/10.1332/204674315X14281321359847

Hussey, D. L., Reed, A. M., Laymann, D. L., & Pasiali, V. (2007). Music therapy and complex trauma: A protocol for developing social reciprocity. *Residential Treatment for Children & Youth, 24*(1–2), 111–129. https://doi.org/10.1300/J007v24n01_07

Kenny, C. (2006). *Music and life in the field of play.* Barcelona Publishers.

Klyve, G. P. (2019). Whose knowledge? Epistemic injustice and challenges in hearing children's voices. *Voices: A World Forum for Music Therapy, 19*(3).

Klyve, G. P., & Rolvsjord, R. (2022). Moments of fun: Narratives of children's experiences of music therapy in mental health care. *Nordic Journal of Music Therapy, 32*(2), 100–120. https://doi.org/10.1080/08098131.2022.2055114

Klyve, G. P., Rolvsjord, R., & Elgen, I. B. (2023). Polyphonic perspectives: A focus group study of interprofessional staff's perceptions of music therapy at an inpatient unit for children in mental health care. *International Journal of Qualitative Studies on Health and Well-Being, 18*(1), 2197750. https://doi.org/10.1080/17482631.2023.2197750

Koelsch, S. (2015). Music-evoked emotions: Principles, brain correlates, and implications for therapy. *Annals of the New York Academy of Sciences, 1337*, 193–201. https://doi.org/10.1111/nyas.12684

Krüger, V. (2019). Music as a structuring resource in identity formation processes by adolescents engaging in music therapy—A case story from a Norwegian child welfare setting. In K. McFerran, P. Derrington, & S. Saarikallio (Eds.), *Handbook of music, adolescents, and wellbeing*. Oxford University Press.

Lave, J., & Wenger, E. (1991). *Situated learning: Legitimate peripheral participation*. Cambridge University Press.

Malloch, S., & Trevarthen, C. (Eds.). (2009). *Communicative musicality: Exploring the basis of human companionship* (pp. 357–376). Oxford University Press.

Malone, K., Tesar, M., & Arndt, S. (2020). *Theorising posthuman childhood studies*. Springer.

Marx, K. (1867/1990). *Capital: A critique of political economy* (B. Fowkes, Trans., Vol. 1). Penguin Books. (Original work published 1867).

Masten, A. S., & Tellegen, A. (2012). Resilience in developmental psychopathology: Contributions of the project competence longitudinal study. *Development and Psychopathology, 24*(2), 345–361. https://doi.org/10.1017/S095457941200003X

Metell, M. (2019). How we talk when we talk about disabled children and their families: An invitation to queer the discourse. *Voices: A World Forum for Music Therapy, 19*(3). https://doi.org/10.15845/voices.v19i3.2652

Murris, K. (2016). *The posthuman child: Educational transformation through philosophy with picturebooks*. Routledge. https://doi.org/10.4324/9781315714405

Perryman, K., Blisard, P., & Moss, R. (2019). Using creative arts in trauma therapy: The neuroscience of healing. *Journal of Mental Health Counseling, 41*(1), 80–94. https://doi.org/10.17744/mehc.41.1.07

Rolvsjord, R. (2010). *Resource-oriented music therapy in mental health care*. Barcelona Publishers.

Santos, A. D. (2018). Empathy and aggression in group music therapy with teenagers: A descriptive phenomenological study. *Music Therapy Perspectives*. Advance online publication. https://doi.org/10.1093/mtp/miy024.

Scrine, E. (2021). The limits of resilience and the need for resistance: Articulating the role of music therapy with young people within a shifting trauma paradigm. *Frontiers in Psychology, 12*, 600245. https://doi.org/10.3389/fpsyg.2021.600245

Shaw, C. M. (2022). An autoethnographic journey in developing post-ableist music therapy. *Voices: A World Forum for Music Therapy, 22*(1). https://doi.org/10.15845/voices.v22i1.3314

Siegel, D. J. (2012). *The developing mind: How relationships and the brain interact to shape who we are* (3rd ed.). Guilford Press.

Sokira, J., Allen, J., & Wagner, H. (2023). The resilience framework for trauma-informed music therapy. In L. Beer & J. C. Birnbaum (Eds.), *Trauma-informed music therapy* (pp. 9–18). Routledge.

Stige, B. (2002). *Culture-centered music therapy.* Barcelona Publishers.

Stige, B., & Aarø, L. E. (2012). *Invitation to community music therapy.* Routledge.

Strehlow, G. (2009). The use of music therapy in treating sexually abused children. *Nordic Journal of Music Therapy, 18*(2), 167–183. https://doi.org/10.1080/08098130903062397

Substance Abuse and Mental Health Services Administration [SAMHSA]. (2014). *SAMHSA's concept of trauma and guidance for a trauma-informed approach.* HHS Publication No. (SMA) 14–4884. Author.

Toader, C., Tataru, C. P., Florian, I. A., Covache-Busuioc, R. A., Bratu, B. G., Glavan, L. A., Bordeianu, A., Dumitrascu, D. I., & Ciurea, A. V. (2023). Cognitive crescendo: How music shapes the brain's structure and function. *Brain Sciences, 13*(10), 1390. https://doi.org/10.3390/brainsci13101390

United Nations. (1989). *Convention on the rights of the child.* https://www.ohchr.org/en/instruments-mechanisms/instruments/convention-rights-child

Viega, M. (2016). Exploring the discourse in hip-hop and implications for music therapy practice. *Music Therapy Perspectives, 34*(2), 138–146. https://doi.org/10.1093/mtp/miv035

Vygotsky, L. (1978). *Mind in society: The development of higher psychological processes.* Harvard University Press.

Weber, M. (1978). In G. Roth & C. Wittich (Eds.), *Economy and society: An outline of interpretive sociology.* University of California Press.

Winnicott, D. W. (2005). *Playing and reality* (2nd ed.). Routledge.

Wyness, M. G. (2012). *Childhood and society: An introduction to the sociology of childhood.* Palgrave Macmillan. https://doi.org/10.1007/978-0-230-24182-4

Zanders, M. L. (2015). Music therapy practices and processes with foster-care youth: Formulating an approach to clinical work. *Music Therapy Perspectives, 33*(2), 97–107.

PART II

Twenty-First-Century Research Supporting Music Therapy and the Best Interest of the Child

CHAPTER 4

Music Therapy in Family and Alternative Care

Introduction

Relevant articles of the Convention on the Rights of the Child (UNCRC) dealing with family and alternative care

Parental guidance and the child's evolving capacities (Article 5): The State must respect the rights and responsibilities of parents and the extended family to provide guidance for the child, which is appropriate to her or his evolving capacities.

Separation from parents (Article 9): The child has a right to live with his or her parents, unless this is deemed to be incompatible with the child's best interests. The child also has the right to maintain contact with both parents if separated from one or both.

Family reunification (Article 10): Children and their parents have the right to leave any country and to enter their own for purposes of reunion or the maintenance of the child–parent relationship.

(*continued*)

V. Krüger, K. M. Murphy, *Child-Centred Music Therapy*,
https://doi.org/10.1007/978-3-031-85724-9_4

(continued)

Parental responsibilities (Article 18): Parents have joint primary responsibility for raising the child, and the State shall support them in this. The State shall provide appropriate assistance to parents in child-raising.

Protection from abuse and neglect (Article 19): The State shall protect the child from all forms of maltreatment by parents or others responsible for the care of the child, and establish appropriate programmes for the prevention of abuse and the treatment of victims.

Protection of a child without a family (Article 20): The State is obliged to provide special protection for a child deprived of the family environment and to ensure that appropriate alternative family care or institutional placement is available in such cases. Efforts to meet this obligation shall pay due regard to the child's cultural background.

Adoption (Article 21): In countries where adoption is recognized and/or allowed, it shall only be carried out in the best interest of the child, and then only with the authorization of competent authorities, and safeguards for the child.

Family Care

Professionally supported family care involves providing families with access to professional services and resources to enhance their ability to care for their children effectively. This support can include counselling, parenting education, health services, and financial assistance, helping families address challenges that may impact their ability to provide a stable and nurturing environment. Music therapy with families is gaining attention for its flexible, holistic approach, using methods like improvisation, instrument play, and musical games (Cobbett, 2016; Tuomi et al., 2021). Sessions often involve not only families but also individuals from their social circles, fostering creative connections (Nicholson et al., 2008). Music therapists often assess family strengths and needs, contributing strategies to treatment plans (Pasiali, 2017). Research suggests that engaging in music therapy strengthens parent–child bonds, improves well-being, and supports emotional and social development while reducing stress and anxiety (Jacobsen & McKinney, 2015; Oldfield, 2017). Typically, music therapists working with families emphasize that the work is tailored to meet the needs of the children in terms of the theoretical approaches that inform their work and the methods that are included in sessions (Edwards, 2011; McIntyre, 2009). Moreover, music therapy researchers have demonstrated the efficacy of music therapy to support children through engagement in music experiences designed to develop the ability to co-regulate and facilitate the parent–child bonds (Guerriero & Blank, 2018).

Research findings and clinical reports suggest that music therapy can improve well-being and health, including improved attachment, engagement, interaction, responsiveness, and sensitivity between parent and child (Teggelove et al., 2019). Music therapy with families can also positively influence children and parents individually including developing better social, emotional, and cognitive skills in the child as well as reducing stress, anxiety, and depression (Gold et al., 2004).

US-based music therapist Kathleen Eberle Cotter works from a systems perspective of music therapy when working with families. Improvisation is a key method in her work.

Kathryn: I often invite families to improvise instrumentally together to observe and later address the structure of the family, patterns of family interaction, family roles, and behaviour as communication. Improvisation allows for exploration between horizontal relationships, such as siblings, and vertical relationships, such as parents to children. It allows for the building of trust as a resource that enables relational partners to give to each other and interact in a healthy manner (as cited in Hargrave & Pfitzer, 2003*). During an initial music therapy session, all family members are invited to select an instrument from a variety of options, with a simple instruction to play together. I observe relational dynamics such as who did everyone look to before the music began? Who played first? Who played the loudest/softest? Who kept a steady beat? Was anyone "doing their own thing", disconnected from the collective sound? Was anyone not participating? Were any members hypervigilant? Did anyone have difficulty not talking during the music? Following the experience, I have a wealth of observations I can genuinely and curiously ask questions about. Questions could be broad, like what was your experience of that music? What sensations did you have in your body while you were playing? What emotions were you feeling during that music? Who could you most clearly hear? How did you know when the music was over? Questions could also be more direct, such as "I noticed Mom got everything started and then kept a steady beat.*

(*continued*)

(continued)
Does Mom play a similar role in your family? I noticed that brother didn't start playing until after everyone else and his music was quiet. Brother, what is it like for you to assert yourself or insert your opinions? I noticed Dad's sound was loud and disconnected. It seemed like you struggled to connect to the beat sometimes. When do you feel disconnected from what is going on at home?" Family members are encouraged to share observations about other members of the family. It is important that during this process, the therapist is not attempting to guide any member to a specific conclusion but is genuinely sharing their own observations and being authentically curious about the interpersonal dynamics made evident in the music. After an improvisation and discussion, I typically facilitate another improvisation with more instruction. Any instruction would be based on the needs or desired changes identified by the family. If the family identified that they struggled to really listen to each other, then I invite the family to listen more closely to how their individual sound fits with everyone else's sound and to be sure they can hear every group member (Cotter & Krüger, in press).

Music Therapy and Families Experiencing Trauma

There is a paucity of research and clinical reports related to the provision of music therapy to children who have been abused or witnessed abuse in their families of origin or alternative care placements. In reviewing the scant literature, we notice several common themes among authors that support the use of music therapy to help family members process these traumatic experiences.

Music therapists work with families in crisis to help them process grief, trauma, and loss, and to develop coping mechanisms for stress and anxiety. Music therapy can provide comfort and hope during difficult times. The literature on family music therapy for children who have experienced trauma emphasizes the importance of helping them co-regulate and reconnect parent-child bonds. Guerriero and Blank (2018) note that "intentional music-making offers parents and children the opportunity to play together." Similarly, Fairchild and Sheridan (2018) state that "in order to create change in children's lives we need to include their family and supportive systems wherever possible" (p. 10). They view music therapy as a means to "create a therapeutic web that invites any healthy and invested people in the child's life to help provide therapeutic opportunities for the child to flourish in the face of adversity" (p. 10).

Lastly, music therapy in family care can be used to amplify the voices of the family members in advocating for their children. Amplifying voices through family care implies speaking out on behalf of families and promoting policies and practices that support family well-being. This practice plays a critical role in ensuring that families have access to the resources and supports they need to thrive. Fairchild and Sheridan (2018) describe a collaborative approach in which they work with children and their nonviolent family members for the purpose of bringing families back together after relationships have been disrupted due to family violence. Music therapy, in their view, can become an important collaborative approach in working creatively with children, young people, and their nonviolent family members as a way of bringing families back together after their relationships have been disrupted due to family violence (Fairchild & Sheridan, 2018).

Fairchild and Sheridan (2018) describe their work in a family setting as a way of bringing families back together after their relationships have been disrupted due to family violence. In this work it became important to establish safety in the initial sessions.

The family sessions provide a space to process their shared experiences, to reflect on the challenges they had experienced, and to share their hopes for the future. The individual sessions provided an opportunity to reflect on their personal experiences and to identify individual strengths and needs. While the family appreciated the space to have their own individual sessions, they eventually decide to continue the therapeutic process as a family and for the remainder of the sessions to be together. Throughout the therapeutic process, a range of creative methods were used to support them to process their experiences, including song-sharing, using picture cards to represent their experiences, drawing their past and present selves, song writing, and musical improvisation to explore their feelings and coping strategies. A significant part of the family's journey was writing a song together in the music therapy sessions. After discussing possibilities for what they could write about, they decided that they wanted to write a song about looking towards a better and bright future and moving on from the past. The family

(*continued*)

(continued)
participated in a typical songwriting process of brainstorming ideas, developing song lyrics, creating a melody and recording the song, which occurred over several sessions. The process of writing the song provided a way for them to work together, to negotiate ideas and to ensure that all voices were represented in the song lyrics.

The old days are long gone

And we are finally moving on

Skies are clearing and we are flying free

Better, brighter times we will see

No more bad dreams No more fear

We're running towards freedom

No more worries No more pain

We're healing from our past

We will be safe We will be free

We will not lose hope

We will laugh again

We will dream

We're looking towards the stars (pp. 8–9)

Alternative Care

Research and clinical reports on the use of music therapy for children in alternative care settings are limited. However, the narrow literature available identifies several recurring themes that advocate for the effectiveness of music therapy in helping these children process their traumatic experiences.

Alternative care includes a range of settings including foster care, residential care, kinship care, and aftercare. This support is provided by social workers, therapists, and other professionals who work closely with caregivers, such as foster parents or guardians, to meet the child's needs and promote their overall well-being in a stable and supportive setting. Even though the main goal of child welfare work is to support the child in living with their biological family, statistically, some cases end up being classified as out-of-home care (Munro, 2011). Being placed in an out-of-home care setting will in many ways interfere with fundamental aspects of a child's life regarding factors such as health and identity (Dovran et al., 2012). Hence, developmental issues such as relationships with parents and friends, school, leisure, health, and education are affected in numerous ways in relation to out-of-home care (Lehmann et al., 2013).

The UN Guidelines for the Alternative Care of Children (2009) outline the need for relevant policy and practice with respect to two basic principles: necessity and appropriateness. The Guidelines for the Alternative Care of Children aims to ensure that children are not placed in alternative care unnecessarily; and that where alternative care is provided, it is delivered under appropriate conditions responding to the rights and best interests of the child (UN, 2009). In particular,

> Financial and material poverty, or conditions directly and uniquely imputable to such poverty, should never be the only justification for the removal of a child from parental care [...] but should be seen as a signal for the need to provide appropriate support to the family. (para. 15)

Foster Care

A foster home is a private home that cares for children who cannot live with their parents. Children in foster care may live with relatives or with unrelated foster parents. Foster parents cooperate with the child protection service in the municipality, and in most cases with the child's family, regarding the child's needs and the child's future. Music therapy in foster care helps children navigate transitions, build relationships, and process emotions through activities like improvisation and songwriting (Zanders et al., 2018; Konieczna-Nowak, 2023). Music therapists working within this field play an important role in finding methods that can help to create relationships in the transition between homes, facilities, schools, and biological families (Wilhelmsen & Fuhr, 2018). Additionally, participation in music therapy can help to create networks and process relationships. Austin (2007) describes working with foster-care youth and notes that "clinical work with adolescents requires a high degree of self-awareness and self-observation because adolescents can 'push buttons' in areas where a therapist is most vulnerable" (p. 102). She reminds us that we as music therapists need working models that give us an understanding of how we should deal with our own difficult emotions when handling adolescents suffering from trauma.

Foster care youth use music as a psychological and social resource. Zanders (2012) noted that foster care youth used simple listening to music:

As a way to calm themselves… [foster care youth] choose music to relax or "chill," either by themselves or with others; as a way to escape from the stressors and difficulties they faced regularly and sometimes to escape from the people who caused them distress; [as a way] to meet a metaphorical and literal need for them to have their own solitary space; as a distraction, which helped to divert their attention away from their mental turmoil or worries; as a way to forget the past. It helped them to forget, neglect, or banish difficult or upsetting thoughts. It may have even helped them avoid dealing with memories or upsetting thoughts, as a catalyst for socialization and identity formation. Listening to music with friends provided these adolescents with an opportunity to discuss and debate life issues, thereby comparing their own perspectives to those of others. This, in turn, helped them to find themselves and shape their own musical and personal identities. (pp. 97–98)

Stuart (2018) demonstrated how music therapy can function as a valuable tool for working with "vulnerable children who have experienced trauma and neglect, working intimately to draw out their playfulness and resilience and create the experience of a safe and trusting relationship." She describes music therapy's role in a case called "Charlie." The case highlights the benefit of music therapy in "all aspects of foster care and the need for collaboration with social welfare systems in under-resourced communities in South Africa."

In the context of South Africa, opportunities to shift with our clients' contexts are rare and often difficult due to limited resources in terms of the small number of music therapists, the lack of awareness of music therapy, and the lack of music therapy posts in the government and social development sectors. It is in the midst of the overburdened South African child welfare system that music therapists could potentially make valuable contributions through collaborations with social workers, child-care workers, funders, and other role-players in the welfare and foster care systems. In the case of Charlie, the collaboration among the POS, the care manager, his foster parent and me, allowed for the provision of therapeutic support through his transition. Music was used to bridge the gap between therapy and community, which was in the case of Charlie, his new foster family. These collaborations may bring about awareness of the psychosocial support that music therapists offer not only to the children in foster care, but also to the under-resourced organizations, social workers, and potential foster parents individuals who attempt to meet the emotional and social needs of children in the foster care system (Stuart, 2018, p. 6).

Music Therapy and Adoption

In context of work with adoption, Article 21 in the UNCRC (1989) emphasizes that adoption, particularly international adoption, must prioritize the best interests of the child, authorized by competent authorities with necessary safeguards. This issue is critical, especially for children from developing countries, as their rights can be compromised when emotional and psychological needs are overlooked in the adoption process. The removal from familiar environments may lead to feelings of loss and identity confusion, affecting their ability to integrate into new families. Despite music therapy's potential to address these emotional challenges, there is limited research on its application for adoptees. Notably, Gravestock (2021) describes how music therapy can help adopted children manage difficult emotions, develop healthy attachments, and build self-esteem. By providing a safe space for musical expression, music therapy fosters connection and belonging, ultimately supporting adopted children in their unique journeys and enhancing their overall well-being.

Residential Care

Music therapy in child welfare offers a way to support children and teens, creating safe spaces for self-expression, emotional growth, and connection. Activities like songwriting and performing, it helps young people navigate challenges, build resilience, and foster meaningful relationships in a supportive, trauma-informed environment. Typically, residential care programmes are "a type of live-in out-of-home care placement in which staff are trained to work with children and youth whose specific needs are best addressed in a highly structured environment" (Childwelfare.gov., 2019). Residential placements are usually time-limited and offer a higher level of structure and supervision than what can be provided through in-home services.

Despite a growing interest in music therapy within child welfare practice, music therapy practices within these contexts is still under-researched. Most of the research conducted in this field is qualitative interview studies and case studies. For example, Van Rooyen and Dos Santos (2020) explore the experiences of teenagers in a children's home in Pretoria, South Africa, who participated in a community music therapy choir over 16 weekly sessions, culminating in a performance of songs they selected. Data from 14 semi-structured interviews were analysed using interpretative phenomenological analysis, revealing meaningful intrapersonal and interpersonal benefits. Intrapersonal outcomes included discovering their musical voices, accessing inner strength for present and future challenges. Interpersonal benefits included relationship growth, improved social skills, and stronger connections with the broader community. The findings highlight the potential of community music therapy to promote personal and social development among youth living in residential care settings.

From a Norwegian context, Krüger et al. (2018) describe a collaborative community music therapy practice that was implemented in a residential care setting. In their study, nine social workers aged 30–55 from four different child welfare institutions were interviewed on their ideas related to the advantages and disadvantages of music therapy. The interview participants' ideas about the benefits of music therapy circled around four main themes: (a) safety and well-being, (b) relationships and mastery, (c) dealing with complex emotions, and (d) continuity and stability, across situations. Findings show that the social workers' reflections around music therapy correspond with child welfare issues such as trauma-informed care and participation (p. 8). Moreover, Krüger et al. (2024) explored challenges and possibilities as expressed by individuals who participated in music workshop facilitated by a music therapist. The participants in the workshop had a background as residents in child protection institutions. The music activities they reported on took place in a public "cultural house" and included listening to music, songwriting, playing in a band and performing, led by music therapists. The authors suggest that work with this population should follow a person-oriented and community-oriented approach, where the child is empowered to take part in activities in community settings where support can be found from peers and adults. By tailoring musical interventions to the individual's current state, music therapists can help clients navigate their emotional landscapes, fostering resilience and enhancing their overall well-being.

When interviewed about their experiences with the music workshop, the adolescents explained that music therapy can be about performing new identities. Experiences in music therapy can also be shared with others, such as social workers who then can learn more about how young people are feeling:

> For example, I showed that song to my two social workers. I didn't dare tell them that I love them, but I showed them the song they understood it, you know. So, it's easier to tell people how you're feeling. (Krüger et al., 2024, p. 11)

They can also be shared through organizing and participating in a concert:

> Here you get treated like an adult, almost. Recently I said that we don't just do music here at [MWS]. When you come here you work with writing lyrics, you play and have fun. And then adults come and say, 'we have a concert coming up,' and we get a goal. You want to work hard toward the concert, since it's a thing you've never done before. And the goal is there, it becomes a sort of hope. (Krüger et al., 2024, p. 11)

Also from a residential care context, Einarsen et al. (2024) interviewed social workers on their experiences with music therapy, and how music is an integral part of the everyday lives of children with who are refugees and living in a residential care setting. Music may serve as a resource to cope with feelings and establish a dialogue between adolescents and adults. Participating in organized cultural initiatives led by music therapists represents a non-confrontational approach where the young person experiences safety, belonging, and participation. However, the participants in the above-mentioned study highlighted the need for knowledge and systematic competencies. They mentioned that not every social worker incorporates music into their practice; while some incorporate sports, others are more active with cultural initiatives. Financial barriers and a lack of economic resources in using culture were also a concern. They argued that the music therapist can act as a catalyst and supervisor for implementing structures for cultural participation, ensuring that the child welfare institution is supported with the benefits of cultural activities.

Work with residential care is often age-specific, and some scholars advocate that specific musical genres are more suitable than others in trying to reach young individuals in residential settings (Viega, 2011). Sullivan (2003) described how hip-hop can be a popular genre among many young people living at an institution. Many may experience the content of this music and culture as negatively charged. At the same time, it is important to understand that one reason that adolescents embrace this music is that their own life story can often be experienced as being as uncensored as the music itself (p. 115). Young people can be encouraged to talk about their experiences related to survival, strength, and suffering by reflecting on and discussing the lyrical content of hip-hop songs (Alvarez, 2012). Similarly, Viega (2016) explored the discourse of hip-hop culture within the context of music therapy. He advocates for the inclusion of hip-hop within music therapy encouraging music therapists to take reflexive positions on "issues such as the cultural appropriation of hip-hop's artistic elements and the manifestation of power and privilege within its musical and therapeutic relationships." According to Viega, learning how to express a certain music genre can be important for one's own identity. However, it seems reasonable to believe that we as music therapists should not be too focused on one genre at the expense of others.

Music Therapy with Families and Alternative Care
Communication and bonding: Music therapy provides situations for family members to connect and express themselves. Music therapy can also help to reduce conflict and build trust.

Increased emotional regulation: Music therapy can help families to manage their emotions in a healthy way. It can also provide a safe space for families to express difficult feelings.

Enhanced coping skills: Music therapy can help families to develop effective coping mechanisms for dealing with stress, anxiety, and trauma. Music therapy can also provide a sense of hope and resilience.

Improved self-esteem and self-awareness: Music therapy can help family members to develop a positive self-image and a better understanding of themselves and others.

Strengthened family relationships: Music therapy can help to strengthen family bonds and promote a sense of unity and belonging.

Attending to the voices of family members: Music therapy provides arenas to be heard.

Creating agency through community work: Music therapy enables social networks and relation.

Gaps in the Research

The above literature review reveals numerous benefits and key roles but also highlights several research gaps that merit further exploration. One significant gap is the limited genre-specific exploration beyond hip-hop (Sullivan, 2003; Viega, 2016), which has been studied in therapy with vulnerable youth. The potential of other musical genres to engage youth based on their diverse cultural and personal identities remains underexplored. Future research could focus on how different genres can engage youth in various settings and how therapists can navigate between musical preferences and therapeutic goals.

Much of the research focuses on music therapy in Western contexts, with limited studies on its application in under-resourced communities or non-Western settings (Stuart, 2018). More cross-cultural research could provide insights into how music therapy practices can be adapted for different cultural backgrounds and socioeconomic conditions, especially in international or multicultural care settings. Music therapy literature emphasizes a holistic and flexible approach, but there is limited research on how cultural differences shape family dynamics and how music therapy interventions should be adapted to respect diverse family structures. Future research could explore culturally tailored interventions, especially in diverse and multicultural settings.

Another gap refers to inconsistent use of music therapy. Research shows that music can play an integral role in supporting adolescents in residential care, especially those who are refugees (Einarsen et al., 2024). However, not all caregivers in family, foster, or residential settings incorporate music into their practice, as some prioritize sports or other cultural activities. More studies could explore the systemic integration of music therapy into residential care and its practical challenges, such as economic barriers and resource constraints.

Moreover, there is limited research on the role of music therapy for children who have been adopted, despite its potential to address issues related to identity, emotional management, and attachment (Gravestock, 2021). Expanding research in this area would help establish a more comprehensive understanding of the unique needs of adoptees in music therapy settings. In foster care settings, while music therapy's role in facilitating transitions and family relationships has been mentioned, it has not been thoroughly studied. Similarly, although trauma-informed care is recognized, research on applying different trauma-informed models within music therapy remains limited. Models like Zanders' (2012) three-stage framework for foster care music therapy lack empirical validation, underscoring the need for more studies to test these frameworks in diverse contexts. Another important area for further investigation is the collaboration between music therapists and other professionals, such as social workers, in care settings. Researching how these partnerships can be optimized through shared decision-making and teamwork may be challenging. Music therapy's potential to facilitate transitions in foster care, such as moving between homes or navigating family relationships, is mentioned but not thoroughly studied (Mandal & Bergset, 2016; Wilhelmsen & Fuhr, 2018). Further investigation into how music therapists can act as "mesoagents" within these transitions could provide clearer frameworks for supporting children's relationships across systems.

Additionally, while the empowering role of music therapy in creating participatory environments for youth has been acknowledged, more robust frameworks for consistently implementing participatory approaches are needed. In family care contexts, there is a notable gap in longitudinal studies assessing the long-term impact of music therapy on family dynamics and child development. Similarly, research on how music therapy interventions can be tailored to different cultural and family structures is lacking. The integration of music therapy with other therapeutic models, such as trauma-informed care or cognitive-behavioural therapy, requires further exploration to understand how these approaches can be effectively combined.

Recommendations for Practice

Music therapy can be a transformative tool for supporting children and families in diverse and challenging environments, particularly in family and alternative care settings. To be effective, music therapists should adopt flexible, holistic, and context-sensitive approaches that consider each family's unique structure and dynamics. This involves incorporating various musical experiences such as improvisation, listening, and shared reflections that align with the cultural and emotional needs of the family. At the heart of these interventions should be a focus on the child's best interest, guided by the UN Convention on the Rights of the Child (UNCRC), which emphasizes fostering positive parent-child relationships, enhancing emotional bonds, and supporting psychological development within a stable family environment.

Music therapists are often part of a professional team. However, more research is needed to understand how music therapy can be better integrated with other therapeutic approaches (e.g. cognitive-behavioural therapy, trauma-informed care) and how these models can be effectively combined in family and alternative care settings. Collaboration with teams, including social workers, counsellors, and teachers, is crucial in providing comprehensive care. Music therapists must communicate their role clearly in assessment and treatment planning, integrating their insights into broader care plans. Families facing trauma, violence, or grief especially benefit from the safe, supportive spaces created by music therapists, where intentional music-making acts as a co-regulation tool, helping family members manage emotions and rebuild connections. Music therapy also serves as a platform for empowerment and advocacy, giving children a voice to express emotions, advocate for their needs, and strengthen relationships within their support networks.

Cultural sensitivity is essential, with therapists tailoring interventions to the diverse sociocultural backgrounds of families, ensuring inclusivity. Additionally, music therapists should incorporate a sociocultural framework in their practice, recognizing the broader influence of schools and communities on a child's development. In alternative care settings such as foster care, ethical considerations must be at the forefront, with interventions aligning with the UN Guidelines for the Alternative Care of Children to ensure necessity and appropriateness. Continuous evaluation and review of interventions are essential to track progress in strengthening family bonds and enhancing children's emotional well-being. Specialized training in trauma-informed care, family dynamics, and professional collaboration is significant for therapists working in these environments, ensuring they are equipped to meet the complex needs of families in crisis. By implementing these practices, music therapists can significantly impact children's and families' well-being, fostering positive emotional and social outcomes in family and alternative care settings.

References

Alvarez, T. T. (2012). Beats, rhymes, and life. Rap therapy in an urban setting. In S. Hadley & G. Yancy (Eds.), *Therapeutic uses of rap and hip-hop* (pp. 117–128). Routledge.

Austin, D. (2007). Lifesongs: Music therapy with adolescents in foster care. In V. Camilleri (Ed.), *Healing the inner-city child: Creative arts therapy with at-risk youth* (pp. 92–103). Jessica Kingsley Publishers.

Cobbett, S. (2016). Context and relationships: Using the systemic approach with music therapy in work with children, adolescents, and their families. *British Journal of Music Therapy, 30*(2), 65–73.

Cotter, K. E., & Krüger, V. (in press). Music therapy and family systems theory. In M. Viega, A. dos Santos, & B. Wheeler (Eds.), *Music therapy handbook*. Guildford Press.

Dovran, A., Winje, D., Arefjord, K., & Haugland, B. S. M. (2012). Traumatic events and posttraumatic reactions among children and adolescents in out-of-home placement: A 25-year systematic literature review. *Journal of Child and Adolescent Trauma, 5*(1), 6–32. https://doi.org/10.1080/19361521.2012.644654

Edwards, J. (2011). The use of music therapy to promote attachment between parents and infants. *The Arts in Psychotherapy, 38*(3), 190–195.

Einarsen, O. K., Krüger, V., Engebretsen, I. M. S., & Stige, B. (2024). Collaboration between social workers and music therapists in a child welfare context for unaccompanied refugee children: A focus group study. *Voices: A*

World Forum for Music Therapy, 24(3) https://doi.org/10.15845/voices.v24i3.4071

Fairchild, R., & Sheridan, J. (2018). Strengthening bonds between children, young people, and their families after family violence. *Voices: A World Forum for Music Therapy, 18*(4), 1–13. https://doi.org/10.15845/voices.v18i4.2600

Gold, C., Voracek, M., & Wigram, T. (2004). Effects of music therapy for children and adolescents with psychopathology: A meta-analysis. *Journal of Child Psychology and Psychiatry, 45*(6), 1054–1059.

Gravestock, J. (2021). *Music therapy in adoption and trauma: Therapy that makes a difference after placement*. Jessica Kingsley Publishers.

Guerriero, A., & Blank, C. A. (2018). Music therapy in a parent-child reunification program: Benefits and challenges of implementation. *Voices: A World Forum for Music Therapy, 18*(4, special issue: Music therapy and child welfare).

Hargrave, T. D., & Pfitzer, F. (2003). *The new contextual therapy: Guiding the power of give and take*. Brunner-Routledge.

Jacobsen, S. L., & McKinney, C. H. (2015). A music therapy tool for assessing parent–child interaction in cases of emotional neglect. *Journal of Child and Family Studies, 24*(7), 2164–2173. https://doi.org/10.1007/s10826-014-0022-6

Konieczna-Nowak, L. (2023). Can you hear me now? The potential of trauma-informed and resilience-oriented music therapy in the context of foster care. *Open Journal Systems, 7*, 153–165. https://doi.org/10.17951/PE/2023.7.153-165

Krüger, V., Nordanger, D. Ø., & Stige. (2018). Music therapy: Building bridges between a participatory approach and trauma-informed care in a child welfare setting. *Voices: A World Forum for Music Therapy, 18*(4) https://voices.no/index.php/voices/article/view/2593

Krüger, V., Lexander, H., Fyhn, T. & Klette-Bøhler, K. (2024). Musisk medborgerskap –musikkverksted som tilnærming i forebyggende arbeid for unge, en kvalitativ analyse av kommunalt ansattes erfaringer. *Fontene Forskning*. [Musical citizenship—music workshop as an approach in preventive work for young people, a qualitative analysis of municipal employees' experiences]. (Fontene Research).

Lehmann, S., Havik, O., Havik, T., & Heiervang, E. (2013). Mental disorders in foster children: A study of prevalence, comorbidity, and risk factors. *Child and Adolescent Psychiatry and Mental Health, 7*(39). https://doi.org/10.1186/1753-2000-7-39

Mandal, A. B., & Bergset, L. J. (2016). Musikkterapi for å skape samanheng i fosterbarn sine nettverk. [Music therapy to create a connection between the networks of a child in foster care.] In K. Stens.th, V. Krüger, & S. Fuglestad (Eds.), *I transitt—mellom til og fra: Om musikk og deltagelse i barnevern* (pp. 143–156). Anthology published by the Center for Research in Music and Health. Oslo, Norway: Norwegian Academy of Music.

McIntyre, J. (2009). Interactive family music therapy: Untangling the system. *The Australian and New Zealand Journal of Family Therapy, 30*(4), 260–268. https://doi.org/10.1375/anft.30.4.260

Munro, E. (2011). *Munro review of child protection, final report: A child-centred system*. Department for Education.

Nicholson, J. M., Berthelsen, D., Abad, V., Williams, K., & Bradley, J. (2008). Impact of music therapy to promote positive parenting and child development. *Journal of Health Psychology, 13*(2), 226–238. https://doi.org/10.1177/1359105307086705

Oldfield, A. (2017). The first 'themed' British journal of music therapy: An introduction to music therapy with families. *British Journal of Music Therapy, 31*(1), 5–11. https://doi.org/10.1177/1359457517697808

Pasiali, V. (2017). Families and children at risk. In S. L. Jacobsen & G. Thompson (Eds.), *Music therapy with families: Therapeutic approaches and theoretical perspectives*. Jessica Kingsley.

Stuart, K. (2018). Musical ripples and reflections: The story of Charlie, his music, and his new foster family. *Voices: A World Forum for Music Therapy, 18*(4). https://doi.org/10.15845/voices.v18i4.2886

Sullivan, L. N. (2003). Meet them in the lab: Using hip-hop music therapy groups with adolescents in residential settings. In N. E. Sullivan, E. S. Mesbur, N. C. Lang, D. Goodman, & L. Mitchell (Eds.), *Social work with groups: Social justice through personal, community, and societal change* (pp. 103–116). The Haworth Press, Inc.

Teggelove, K., Thompson, G., & Tamplin, J. (2019). Supporting positive parenting practices within a community-based music therapy group program: Pilot study findings. *Journal of Community Psychology, 47*(4), 712–726. https://doi.org/10.1002/jcop.22148

Tuomi, K., Thompson, G., Gottfried, T., & Ala-Ruona, E. (2021). Theoretical perspectives and therapeutic approaches in music therapy with families. *Voices: A World Forum for Music Therapy, 21*(2). https://doi.org/10.15845/voices.v21i2.2952

United Nations. (1989). *Convention on the rights of the child*. https://www.ohchr.org/en/instruments-mechanisms/instruments/convention-rights-child

United Nations. (2009). *Guidelines for the alternative care of children*. Retrieved from https://digitallibrary.un.org/record/673583?ln=en&v=pdf

Van Rooyen, A., & Dos Santos, A. (2020). Exploring the lived experiences of teenagers in a children's home participating in a choir: A community music therapy perspective. *International Journal of Community Music, 13*(1), Article 00011. https://doi.org/10.1386/ijcm_00011_1

Viega, M. (2011). The hero's journey in hip-hop and its applications in music therapy. In S. Hadley & G. Yancy (Eds.), *Therapeutic uses of rap and hip-hop* (p. 22). Routledge. https://doi.org/10.4324/9780203806012

Viega, M. (2016). Exploring the discourse in hip-hop and implications for music therapy practice. *Music Therapy Perspectives, 34*(2), 138–146. https://doi.org/10.1093/mtp/miv035

Wilhelmsen, C., & Fuhr, G. (2018). Reflections on practice: Three examples of relational music therapy practice with adolescents in child welfare services. *Voices: A World Forum for Music Therapy, 18*(4).

Zanders, M. L. (2012). The musical and personal biographies of adolescents with foster care experience. In *Collected work: Qualitative inquiries in music therapy. VII* (pp. 71–109). Barcelona Publishers.

Zanders, M. L., Midach, M., Waldmeier, L., & Barros, B. (2018). A reflexive music therapy clinical introspection in working with foster care youth. *Voices: A World Forum for Music Therapy, 18*(4).

CHAPTER 5

Music Therapy in Educational and Cultural Contexts

Written by Maren Metell

Introduction

This chapter gives an overview of children's educational and cultural rights in the respective contexts of kindergarten, schools, and cultural activities in the community. The first part of the chapter offers an overview of relevant articles from the UNCRC (1989) and the Convention on the Rights of People with Disabilities (2007), UNCRC comments and other guidelines. The second part focuses on different contexts and settings as primary school and kindergarten and reviews research, policies, and practices to exemplify how these rights are currently addressed and why these rights matter to children.

Relevant articles of the Convention on the Rights of the Child (UNCRC) dealing with educational and cultural rights:

Disabled children's rights to participation (Article 23). "States Parties recognize that a mentally or physically disabled child should enjoy a full and decent life, in conditions which ensure dignity, promote self-reliance and facilitate the child's active participation in the community."

(*continued*)

V. Krüger, K. M. Murphy, *Child-Centred Music Therapy*,
https://doi.org/10.1007/978-3-031-85724-9_5

(continued)

Right to education (Article 28). "States Parties recognize the right of the child to education, and with a view to achieving this right progressively and on the basis of equal opportunity (...)."

Aim of education (Article 29). "States Parties agree that the education of the child shall be directed to the development of the child's personality, talents and mental and physical abilities to their fullest potential, b) the development of respect for human rights and freedoms, the respect of the child's parents, cultural identity, languages and values, c, the preparation of the child for responsible life in a free society."

Right to leisure, play and culture (Article 31). "1. States Parties recognize the right of the child to rest and leisure, to engage in play and recreational activities appropriate to the age of the child and to participate freely in cultural life and the arts. 2. States Parties shall respect and promote the right of the child to participate fully in cultural and artistic life and shall encourage the provision of appropriate and equal opportunities for cultural, artistic, recreational and leisure activity."

Music is thus a right enshrined in both the UNCRC and UNCRPD (UN Committee on the Rights of Persons with Disabilities) which is linked to other rights such as education and participation. While some countries have not ratified either of these, there is a focus internationally on the importance of having access to music. Children with disabilities often become music therapy participants, because they have the right for support based on a diagnosis. As all other children, disabled children have their rights recognized in the UNCRC. Additionally, their rights are enshrined in the CRPD which adds a focus on the specific situation of disabled children. For instance, while the UNCRC recognizes the rights of children to participate in cultural life (Article 31), the CRPD adds a perspective on access on equal basis with others to cultural life (Article 30). Thus, the conventions overlap and complement each other.

Relevant articles of the Convention on the Rights of People with Disabilities dealing with educational and cultural rights

Children with disabilities (Article 7). "States Parties shall take all necessary measures to ensure the full enjoyment by children with disabilities of all human rights and fundamental freedoms on an equal basis with other children."

Accessibility (Article 9). "To enable persons with disabilities to live independently and participate fully in all aspects of life, States Parties shall take appropriate measures to ensure to persons with disabilities access, on an equal basis with others, to the physical environment, to transportation, to information and communications, including information and communications technologies and systems, and to other facilities and services open or provided to the public, both in urban and in rural areas."

Education (Article 24). "States Parties recognize the right of persons with disabilities to education. With a view to realizing this right without discrimination and on the basis of equal opportunity, States Parties shall ensure an inclusive education system at all levels and lifelong learning (…)."

Participation in cultural life, recreation, leisure and sport (Article 30). "States Parties recognize the right of persons with disabilities to take part on an equal basis with others in cultural life, and shall take all appropriate measures to ensure that persons with disabilities: (a) Enjoy access to cultural materials in accessible formats; (b) Enjoy access to television programmes, films, theatre and other cultural activities, in accessible formats; (c) Enjoy access to places for cultural performances or services, such as theatres, museums, cinemas, libraries and tourism services, and, as far as possible, enjoy access to monuments and sites of national cultural importance."

Disabled children often experience barriers to participation in music. These barriers include, as for other activities, lack of accessibility of venues, assistive technology, access to transportation as well as attitudes towards disability (UN, 2013). The UN CRC Committee (2013) commented on Article 31 emphasizing the importance of play for children's well-being and points to groups of children (including disabled children) that experience barriers. They emphasize that it is important to create "time and space for children to engage in spontaneous play, recreation and creativity, and to promote societal attitudes that support and encourage such activity" (CRC Committee, 2013, p. 3).

As McLaughlin et al. (2016) and Mallett and Runswick (2014) point out, disabled children often experience that play (and we think that applies to music too) becomes into a site for surveillance and intervention. Music (therapy) can therefore have an ambiguous role in the life of disabled children being a right, a leisure activity, and sometimes an activity used by adults for assessment and intervention.

Kindergarten and Preschool Settings

The right to education is a fundamental human right accepted as legally binding by all member states of the United Nations (1989). Music therapy within educational systems, if existent, is organized differently in different parts of the world. We will here review research and aim to give examples from a variety of contexts but know that non-Western and Global South contexts will be underrepresented. Kindergarten, nursery, and preschool are the educational settings children attend in many countries before they enter primary school. As UNESCO and UNICEF (2024) point out, there is no international legal framework guaranteeing children's right to early education. According to UNESCO and UNICEF (2024), almost 60% of children in low-income countries do not have access to preschool education at all. Depending on the context, music may or may not be part of the curriculum. In Finland, the development of children's musical, visual, crafts are one of the tasks for early childhood education (The Finnish National Agency for Education, 2022).

In Norway, for instance, the regulatory framework plan for kindergarten (Utdanningsdirektoratet, 2017) describes "art, culture and creativity" as one of the learning areas kindergartens are supposed to work with. In Portugal, the ministry of education (2024) presents music as one of the approaches to learn if the child is interested in participating in diverse cultural practices and symbolic languages. Music is also part of the curriculum for children between three and six in China (Ministry of Education of the People's Republic of China, 2012) both as art and as means for learning.

Articles 7 and 9 of the CRPD point to disabled children's right to all aspects of life and the accessibility of spaces and arenas. Vatnedalen Vik et al. (2023) focus on the possibilities of "including all" through singing. They argue that facilitating musical meeting spaces in kindergarten creates preconditions for communication and interaction for all children, especially those that have needs for adaptions.

Birch and Thompson (2023) sought to identify key characteristics of music therapy research in preschool settings that include disabled children in their scoping review. The 19 peer-reviewed articles included in the review point out that music therapy practice is informed by funding policies and educational systems. Delivery models include individual- and group-based music therapy and consultation. "Social interaction skills" are identified as a common goal across the articles and the authors wonder if this is related to the mainly US-based projects where behavioural and developmental frameworks are common. Birch and Thomas (2023) point to the possibilities of music therapy in these contexts that often already use music as part of their everyday routines. They emphasize that the location of sessions (as classroom, playground or separate room) can promote or hinder inclusion. The topic of location of music therapy will also be discussed in the subsequent section.

Davies and Rosscornes (2012) provide one concrete example for music therapy practice in educational and day-care settings for preschool children aged three months to four years within a multicultural and socioeconomically diverse community in the UK. They describe the provision of music therapy as music therapy sessions, drop-in community music groups and singing in the day-care rooms, and ukulele workshops for parents and staff. This example shows the myriad ways in which music therapy can be incorporated into a pre-school setting.

Helle-Valle et al. (2017) explore the topic of children's restlessness in a Norwegian pre-school setting. They argue that community music therapy "can be useful when working towards enhanced mutual relationships between the individual and his or her ecological system" (p. 13). Community music therapy is presented as a framework that makes adult and systemic contributions to children's restlessness visible and restlessness as a process. The examples provided in this section show different approaches and foci in pre-school settings and point to the potential of music therapy to facilitate young children's rights to music and participation.

Music Therapy in Inclusive School Settings

The extent to which children have access to music therapy varies among countries. Further, as noted by McFerran and Crooke (2014), there are significant gaps in practices even when music therapy is provided. Music therapists that work in school settings focus on a broad range of goal areas such as developmental goals (Jordan et al., 2018), facilitating musical participation (Parsons, 2022) violence prevention (Wölfl, 2014) and creating music cultures (Rickson & McFerran, 2014). Music therapy may be provided to a diverse group of students including children with disabilities (e.g. Hayes, 2016), emotional/behavioural challenges (Chong & Kim, 2010), or from a refugee background (e.g. Enge & Stige, 2022; Hunt, 2005). Additionally, music therapists provide consultation services (Rickson, 2012). Music therapy projects have also taken place in schools in response to catastrophes (e.g. bushfires in Australia, McFerran & Teggelove, 2011) and to address global challenges such as dropout (Krüger et al., 2024).

The focus in this section is on school settings that are depending on context called local, regular, or mainstream schools. Carr and Wigram (2009) carried out a systemic review on music therapy in mainstream schools including background and policy data from the UK. The authors don't define the term "mainstream school" but exclude studies of children with complex support needs as they describe that these often receive music therapy that occur outside school (which might be different in many other contexts). Their findings point to the usefulness of music therapy in school settings pointing to its affordances for social and emotional needs, but also to the need for more research.

Using a descriptive phenomenological design, dos Santos (2018) discusses the therapeutic potential of group music therapy for adolescents referred for aggression. She highlights how music therapy groups provide a safe space where adolescents can express and explore their aggression, alongside feelings of pain, loneliness, fear, and guilt. In this context, aggression begins to lose its legitimacy and meaning as the participants experience support, trust, safety, and validation—not only from the music therapist but also from their peers. Through various forms of musicking such as songwriting and improvisation, the adolescents can process these complex emotions while simultaneously being exposed to positive relational dynamics. Similarly, by further exploring group music therapy through, Santos (2019) highlighted the importance of a client-centred approach that balances structure and freedom while considering empathy in diverse ways. Drawing on Deleuze's (1990) and Gergen's (2009) theories, she emphasizes the usefulness of understanding aggression within a non-judgemental music therapy setting. In this study key implications for practice included a more inclusive view of empathy, and the importance of considering various therapeutic assemblages.[1]

Rickson's (2012) research contributes to the body of evidence that supports music therapy's role in school settings, encouraging music therapists to consider providing support to teachers and other professionals rather than working directly with students in inclusive settings. Rickson (2012) analysed four case studies and developed a protocol consisting of following consultation stages: establishing therapeutic relationships, collaborative assessment and goal setting, implementation of music strategies, and follow-up and evaluation. Rickson's approach to consultation can be linked to Article 24 of the CRPD, pointing to the right to inclusive education.

The UNCRPD and the right to inclusive education have contributed to more music therapy in schools in German-speaking countries (Lutz Hochreutener, 2018). To not discriminate against disabled children, pedagogical settings consequently need to be inclusive and facilitate access to music, Lutz Hochreutener argues. Discussing challenges and chances Lutz Hochreutener points to the differences between the fields of education and therapy in terms of space, goals, time frame, attitudes, rules and values, but also advocates for interdisciplinary dialogue. Further, Lutz Hochreutener positions the low threshold for children receiving support in a space that they spend a lot of time in.

Pethybridge and Robertson (2010) use the term "educational music therapy" to describe their approach to working in a school setting. They argue that "once children are contributing to the music-making environment within a school context and taking ownership of their own musical interaction in small groups, they can become more available to address

[1] The following is a definition on what an assemblage is based on Deleuze and Parnet "What is an assemblage? It is a multiplicity which is made up of many heterogeneous terms and which establishes liaisons, relations between them, across ages, sexes and reigns—different natures" (Deleuze and Parnet, Dialogues II, p. 69).

educational objectives, both musical and non-musical" based on their experiences in the educational setting (Pethybridge & Robertson, 2010, p. 142).

Rickson and McFerran (2014) base their book *Creating Music Culture in Schools* on the premise that "all young people have a right to participate meaningfully and authentically in their school community and therefore have a need for the unique conditions afforded by music" (p. 13). In their musical tree fig. (2014, p. 14), they share their vision of flourishing, sustainable music cultures in schools:

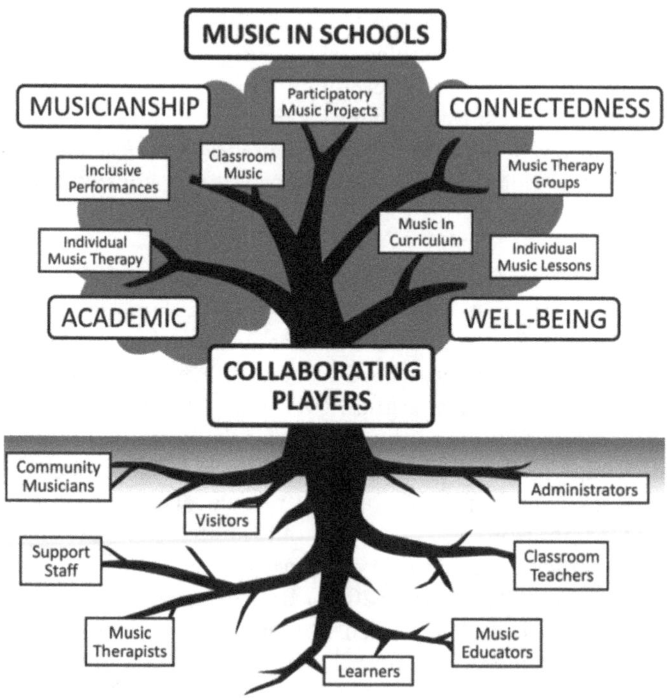

The roots represent the different human actors that get music into action in school. The trunk displays these actors as collaborating players. The treetop consists of different affordances, such as connectedness and well-being. The branches are practices and structures (classroom music, inclusive affordances, individual and group music therapy). While non-human actors as artefacts are missing in the picture, it visualizes a vision of a flourishing music culture in a complex system.

Parsons (2022), exploring aspects of power and language, describes her various ways in being involved with music culture in music therapy practice within mainstream primary schools (UK). Parsons is employed as music therapist and teacher and describes her role as follows:

My dual role as both music teacher and music therapist connects me with all the school's students and staff. I am, therefore, able to observe various musical practices, how they distribute throughout the school, and how they affect those involved. For example, in my work, I may see a child individually on a weekly basis and engage in song writing. I then may see this child raise their hand in a whole-class music lesson when asked if anyone has ever written a song. Or, I may see this child engaging in song writing with a friend during their break time. (...)

In my own work, I have been called the music therapist, the music teacher, the music lady, and the music person. The music room has been called a therapeutic space, a teaching space, a fun space, and a safe space. Musical action has been labelled therapeutic, educational, enjoyable, and calming. These language choices are made day-to-day by children, their families, and our staff. Musicking comes from several practices including and not including me. Of importance is the connection of these practices. The child who writes a song in her music lesson doesn't compartmentalize that experience to an education box. She shares it in her everyday life and relocates its origins in other times and spaces and, thus, ecologies are built.

The ecology of the setting of the school in Parson's (2022) example affords rich possibility across settings, whereas in other contexts this type of collaboration seems to challenge values and practices. Collaboration is also necessary in research to make sure all voices are heard. As an example, Devlin et al. (2024) collaborated with Morgan, a teenager with Down syndrome, and Chery, Morgan's mother, to explore their shared experience of music therapy in the school setting and the music therapy clinic (Devlin et al., 2024). The school setting impacted their music therapeutic work by supporting their values of "following rules" and "fitting in." At the clinic, Morgan could use music to express herself and making mistakes was fine. Similarly, Mössler et al. (2023) described how the school context challenged what the music therapists would think was acceptable to do within the music therapy room. A video clip showing an autistic child exploring the sound of Lego bricks, was identified by the music therapist as a moment of failed attunement as they felt unsure about how to engage with the child's activity. Trying to engage musically with the child in different ways, the music therapist didn't feel capable. This was the starting point for the exploration of attunement dynamics between the autistic child and the non-autistic music therapist. The music therapist and focus group participants identified the expectations and norms linked to the school setting as framing what happened in music therapy.

These different examples show that there is a tension between education and therapy in many contexts and point to sometimes conflicting approaches and values. However, there are also several examples making the affordances of music therapy visible on individual, group, and systemic levels.

Music Therapy in Non-inclusive School Settings

Music and music therapy have in many countries a long tradition in non-inclusive school settings (e.g. Nordoff & Robbins, 1971) as schools or departments that serve exclusively disabled children. In their comment on Article 24, the UN committee presents their concerns about the challenges that persist, denying disabled children their rights and access to inclusive education.

> Ensuring the right to inclusive education entails a transformation in culture, policy and practice in all formal and informal educational environments to accommodate the differing requirements and identities of individual students, together with a commitment to removing the barriers that impede that possibility. It involves strengthening the capacity of the education system to reach out to all learners. It focuses on the full and effective participation, accessibility, attendance and achievement of all students, especially those who, for different reasons, are excluded or at risk of being marginalized. (UN, 2016, General comment No. 4 on Article 24)

For the past 30 years there have been international initiatives to encourage inclusive education that makes a quality educational available to all learners (Ainscow, 2020). Despite these initiatives, children with support needs are segregated in different forms of schools or classes in many countries.

Music therapists in non-inclusive settings often work in close collaboration with teachers and other professionals, based on the goals in a student's individual educational plan. In other schools, music therapists are considered health professionals and work more independently in goals that are not necessarily part of an individual plan. They also can work on system level, providing supervision or consultation work (Rickson, 2012).

Music therapists in non-inclusive school settings engage students in music experiences to address a wide range of goals, communication being a central one (e.g. Elefant, 2010; McFerran & Stephenson, 2010). Elefant (2010) describes her work in a "special education centre" in Israel, working as a member of the interdisciplinary team. Together with girls with Rett syndrome and their families, she researched the capacity of songs in music therapy to enhance communicative abilities. Their results show that the children could communicate song choices, learn, and sustain learning over time. McFerran and Stephenson (2010) conducted a study on the benefits of individual music therapy for developing communication skills for student's complex support needs. They compared the number of communicative acts the students produced during music therapy as compared when interacting with the music therapist in the absence of music. Statistical measures using conventional communication measures could not show a clear difference in communicative acts between music therapy and nonmusical play with the same music therapist. However, a qualitative exploration of the same video footage identifies four principles of musical engagement and emphasizes the importance of experiences of relationships (McFerran & Shoemark, 2013).

Music therapists working in non-inclusive settings can, just as in other school settings, experience tension between their own approach and the system they work in. On the one hand, they are attempting to create a more anti-oppressive space, while also having to deal with resistance as, for instance, having passed down restrictions on the use of stimming toys or certain music genres (Metell & Leza, 2023).

Similarly, Shaw and Metell (in press) point to the responsibility of music therapists to work collaboratively with children to develop goals and activities in music therapy together. The authors recommend moving away from normative goals that may be ableist and towards developing goals and focus areas together with music therapy participants. Music therapists can thus have an important role in ensuring (disabled) children's access to music and defending their rights for participation and play.

The Right to Music and Music Therapy in Cultural Contexts

The International Music Council (n.d.) developed the five music rights, first proclaimed in Tokyo in 2001 which are inspired by the Universal Declaration of Human Rights and the Declaration of the Rights of the Child. The first three of these apply to children and adults, stating that they have the right to express themselves musically, to learn musical language and skills and to have access to musical involvement.

Article 30 of the UNCRC and Article 31 of the UNCRPD point to the cultural rights of all children. Children need to have access to music early in life to be able to use music to the fullest capacity later in life (Curtis & Vaillancourt, 2012).

Music therapists work in different ways depending upon their cultural contexts. This can include adapted instrumental lessons (e.g. Jackson, 2018), facilitation of music workshops (Krüger et al., 2024), and work project/performance oriented (Mitchell, 2019). However, barriers such as physical accessibility and lack of transport and accessible information often hinder participation in cultural events and leisure activities (The Civil Society Coalition Norway, 2019, p. 33). In the UK, Creative United's (2018) research showed that 49% of parents reported that their children had moderate to severe limitations when trying to access music lessons. Over 50% of music educators reported that access to suitable instruments was a barrier that impeded their students' ability to participate in music making. In Norway, disabled children and youth have reported that they lack assistance to attend leisure activities as venues and transport are often not accessible. Additionally, they experience to not being listened to (Save the Children, 2021). These are just two examples highlighting the significant gap between the formal rights and current practices of making venues, transport, and information accessible.

Especially in the context of disabled children, it is important to understand music as a right for all children, independently of their support needs. Access to and participation in music and other cultural activities should not be linked to a therapeutical aim. Both music educators and music therapists have questioned that practice of referring disabled children to a music therapist, rather than a music educator (Metell, 2014; Skogdal, 2015). It is important for both music therapists and music educators to be reflexive when considering their roles and competences in creating inclusive music cultures. Music therapists can play an important role in challenging normative music aesthetics and creating spaces for more inclusive musical participation. They have a potential to work against barriers. The practice of consultation described above seems to be an important way of practice in cultural contexts too.

Gaps in the Research

Compared to other fields of music therapy, research in educational and leisure settings is scant. The research presented above shows the potential of music therapy on both an individual and institutional level to contribute significantly to ensure that children can exercise their rights to music and participation.

There is, however, a need to collect more evidence of when this happens and how and for whom as, for instance, Parsons (2022) does in a mainstream school. There is a lack of systematic reviews (exemptions are Birch & Thompson, 2023, and Carr & Wigram, 2009) related to music therapy in educational settings as a means of creating a more robust evidence base. Research on music therapy in educational setting in the Global South is limited which leaves us with a fragmented picture of music therapy practice in the international community.

Rickson and McFerran (2014) describe the potential roles music therapists can play in schools. However, there is a need to explore these roles in more depth and in different contexts. As an example, what might the role be of the music therapist in creating more inclusive learning environments for all school age children from pre-school through graduation? How can music therapists work on different levels through direct and indirect work, working with children, their teachers and schools? Finally, the role of music therapy in such settings has yet not adequately been researched.

Articles 12 and 13 of the UNCRC (1989) highlight the importance of listening to and respecting children's experiences. Music therapy can be considered a way to safeguard children's rights to participation, but the majority of music therapy research is still on children rather than with children. From our perspective there is an urgent need for more participatory research with children that focuses on their perspectives (see also the chapter in this book on research).

Recommendations for Practice

We offer the following recommendations for practice to ensure that all children have access to music activities and, if needed, music therapy. From an institutional level, creating structures for employment of music therapists on different levels of organizations, municipalities, and the cultural sector seems a central effort to create more accessible music spaces and ensure that children can perform their rights to music. Regarded from an individual level, music therapists, as all other people working with children, need to reflect and question the structures they work in and then challenge those structures and aspects in their thinking, approaches and that prevent children from exercising their rights to music (Metell, 2023; Metell & Leza, 2023; Rickson & McFerran, 2014). As seen from a systemic level, music therapists can have an important role in making other people aware of (disabled) children's rights to music (Courtis & Vaillancourt, 2012) and to create opportunities where these rights can be exercised. Close collaboration with children, teachers, kindergarten teachers, parents, other professionals, local NGOs, and governmental organizations is necessary to create sustainable music practices (Krüger et al., 2023; The Civil Society Coalition Norway, 2019).

One important aspect of music therapy practice in educational contexts presented above (and we would extend this to cultural contexts) is consultation. To work as a consultant (Rickson, 2012) in kindergartens, schools, and cultural organizations can be a way to increase awareness of children's rights to music and while creating environments where music is accessible. In practice, this might mean providing consultation and continuing education for kindergarten teachers, teachers, social workers, and everyone interested in learning more about making music accessible.

References

Ainscow, M. (2020). Promoting inclusion and equity in education: Lessons from international experiences. *Nordic Journal of Studies in Educational Policy, 6*(1), 7–16. https://doi.org/10.1080/20020317.2020.1729587

Birch, J., & Thompson, G. (2023). Exploring music therapy research in preschool settings that include children with disabilities: A scoping review. *The Journal of Music Therapy, 60*(1), 64–97. https://doi.org/10.1093/jmt/thac015

Carr, C., & Wigram, T. (2009). Music therapy with children and adolescents in mainstream schools: A systematic review. *British Journal of Music Therapy, 23*(1), 3–18. https://doi.org/10.1177/135945750902300102

Chong, H. J., & Kim, S. J. (2016). Education-oriented music therapy as an after-school program for students with emotional and behavioural problems. *The Arts in Psychotherapy, 37*(3), 190–196. https://doi.org/10.1016/j.aip.2010.03.004

Civil Society Coalition Norway. (2019). *Alternative report to the UN Committee on the rights of persons with disabilities.* https://unge-funksjonshemmede.no/rapport-til-fn-funksjonshemmedes-rettigheter-brytes-i-norge/

Curtis, S., & Vaillancourt, G. (2012). The children's right to music project. *Voices: A World Forum for Music Therapy, 12*(3).

Davies, E., & Rosscornes, C. (2012). Setting up and developing music therapy at a children's centre, for pre-school children and their families and carers. In J. Tomlinson, P. Derrington, & A. Oldfield (Eds.), *Music therapy in schools: Working with children of all ages in mainstream and special education* (pp. 19–32). Jessica Kingsley Publishers.

Deleuze, G. (1990). *The logic of sense* (M. Lester & C. Stivale, Trans.). Columbia University Press.

Devlin, K., Johnston, M., & Johnston, C. (2024). Making mistakes together: Therapy participant, parent, and therapist perspectives on music therapy in two different settings. *Music Therapy Perspectives, 42*(2), 129–138. https://doi.org/10.1093/mtp/miae007

dos Santos, A. (2019). Empathy and aggression in group music therapy with teenagers: A descriptive phenomenological study. *Music Therapy Perspectives, 37*(1), 14–27. https://doi.org/10.1093/mtp/miy024

Elefant, C. (2010). Unmasking hidden resources: Communication in children with severe developmental disabilities in music therapy. In V. Karkou (Ed.), *Arts therapies in schools: Research and practice* (pp. 243–258). Jessica Kingsley Publishers.

Enge, K. E. A., & Stige, B. (2022). Musical pathways to the peer community: A collective case study of refugee children's use of music therapy. *Nordic Journal of Music Therapy, 31*(1), 7–24. https://doi.org/10.1080/08098131.2021.1891130

Finnish National Agency for Education. (2022). *National core curriculum for early childhood education and care.* https://www.oph.fi/sites/default/files/documents/Varhaiskasvatussuunnitelman%20perusteet%202022_EN_final_23%20.pdf

Gergen, K. (2009). *Relational being: Beyond self and community*. Oxford University Press.

Hayes, T. (2016). Music therapy in the context of the special school. In J. Edwards (Ed.), *The Oxford handbook of music therapy* (176–185). Oxford University Press.

Helle-Valle, A., Binder, P.-E., Anderssen, N., & Stige, B. (2017). Is restlessness best understood as a process? Reflecting on four boys' restlessness during music therapy in kindergarten. *International Journal of Qualitative Studies on Health and Well-Being, 12*(supl), 1298266–1298215. https://doi.org/10.1080/17482631.2017.1298266

Hunt, M. (2005). Action research and music therapy: Group music therapy with young refugees in a school community. *Voices: A World Forum for Music Therapy, 5*(2). https://doi.org/10.15845/voices.v5i2.223

International Music Council. (n.d.). *Home*. International Music Council. https://imc-cim.org/

Jackson, N. (2018). Therapeutic lessons with a girl with Down syndrome. In A. Heiderscheit & N. Jackson (Eds.), *Introduction to music therapy practice* (pp. 33–39). Barcelona Publishers.

Jordan, A.-K., Pfeifer, E., Stegemann, T., & Lutz Hochreutener, S. (Eds.). (2018). *Musiktherapie in pädagogischen Settings: Impulse aus Praxis*. Theorie und Forschung.

Krüger, V., Crooke, A., Solberg, D., & Sæle, E. (2023). Exploring the potential for music therapy to support 21st century education goals: Interviews with six Norwegian teachers. *Voices: A World Forum for Music Therapy, 23*(1). https://doi.org/10.15845/voices.v23i1.3642

Krüger, V., Lexander, H., Fyhn, T., & Klette-Bøhler, K. (2024). Musisk medborgerskap – musikkverksted som tilnærming i forebyggende arbeid for unge, en kvalitativ analyse av kommunalt ansattes erfaringer. *Fontene Forskning*. [Musical citizenship – Music workshop as an approach in preventive work for young people, a qualitative analysis of municipal employees' experiences. *Fontene Research*].

Lutz Hochreutener, S. (2018). Musiktherapie im schulischen Kontext. Fakten—Herausforderungen—Chancen. In A. Jordan, E. Pfeifer, T. Stegemann, & S. L. Hochreutener (Eds.), *Musiktherapie in pädagogischen Setting. Impulse aus Praxis, Theorie und Forschung* (pp. 15–30).

Mallett, R., & Runswick-Cole, K. (2014). *Approaching disability: Critical issues and perspectives* (1st ed.). Routledge.

McFerran, K. S., & Crooke, A. (2014). Enabling tailored music programs in elementary schools: An Australian exemplar. *Journal of Education and Training Studies, 2*(4). https://doi.org/10.11114/jets.v2i4.536

McFerran, K. S., & Shoemark, H. (2013). How musical engagement promotes well-being in education contexts: The case of a young man with profound and multiple disabilities. *International Journal of Qualitative Studies on Health and Well-Being, 8*, 20570. https://doi.org/10.3402/qhw.v8i0.2057

McFerran, K., & Stephenson, J. (2010). Facing the challenge: A music therapy investigation in the evidence-based framework. In V. Karkou (Ed.), *Arts therapies in schools: Research and practice* (pp. 259–270). Jessica Kingsley Publishers.

McFerran, K. S., & Teggelove, T. (2011). Music therapy with young people in schools: After the Black Saturday fires. *Voices: A World Forum for Music Therapy, 11*(1).

McLaughlin, J., Coleman-Fountain, E., & Clavering, E. (2016). *Disabled childhoods: Monitoring differences and emerging identities* (1st ed.). Routledge. https://doi.org/10.4324/9781315795898

Metell, M. (2014). Disabling musicking: Reflections on a disability studies perspective in music therapy. *Voices: A World Forum for Music Therapy, 14*(3). https://doi.org/10.15845/voices.v14i3.786

Metell, M. (2023). *Disabled children's access to music.* Music's Transform.

Metell, M., & Leza, J. (2023). Exploring queer theories as a framework for anti-oppressive music therapy practice with neurodivergent children and youth. In C. A. Lee (Ed.), *The Oxford handbook of queer and trans music therapy* (pp. 370–385). Oxford University Press. https://doi.org/10.1093/oxfordhb/9780192898364.013.21

Ministry of Education of the People's Republic of China. (2012). *Guideline for learning and development of children aged 3–6.* Beijing, China: Ministry of Education. https://www.unicef.cn/sites/unicef.org.china/files/2018-10/2012-national-early-learning-development-guidelines.pdf),

Mitchell, E. (2019). Community music therapy and participatory performance: Case study of a coffee house. *Voices: A World Forum for Music Therapy, 19*(1). https://doi.org/10.15845/voices.v19i1.2701

Mössler, K., Halstead, J., Metell, M., Gottschewski, K., & Schmid, W. (2023). "The room is a mess": Exploring the co-creation of space for attunement dynamics between an autistic child and a non-autistic music therapist. *Nordic Journal of Music Therapy*, 1–21. https://doi.org/10.1080/08098131.2022.2145346

Nordoff, P., & Robbins, C. (1971). *Music therapy in special education* (p. 253). John Day Company.

Parsons, J. (2022). Whose "power of music"? Questioning and problematizing aspects of language and power in music therapy practice within mainstream primary schools in the UK. *Voices: A World Forum for Music Therapy, 22*(3). https://doi.org/10.15845/voices.v22i3.3406

Pethybridge, E., & Robertson, J. (2010). Educational music therapy: Theoretical foundations explored in time-limited group work projects with children. In V. Karkou (Ed.), *Arts therapies in schools: Research and practice* (pp. 129–144). Jessica Kingsley Publishers.

Rickson, D. (2012). Music therapy school consultation: A unique practice. *Nordic Journal of Music Therapy, 21*(3), 268–285. https://doi.org/10.1080/08098131.2012.654474

Rickson, D., & McFerran, K. (2014). *Creating music cultures in the schools: A perspective from community music therapy.* Barcelona Publishers.

Santos, A. D. (2018). Empathy and aggression in group music therapy with teenagers: A descriptive phenomenological study. *Music Therapy Perspectives.* Advance online publication. https://doi.org/10.1093/mtp/miy024.

Save the children. (2021). *Fritid for alle—uten fordommer. Fortellinger om fritid fra barn og ungdom med funksjonsnedsettelse [Leisure time for everyone –without prejudices. Narratives on leisure time from children and youth with disability].*

Shaw, C., & Metell, M. (in press). Music therapy and disability. In I. B. Wheeler, M. Viega, & A. dos Santos (Eds.), *Music therapy handbook.* Guildford Press.

Skogdal, E. (2015). Hvem får være musikkelev?—Kunstdidaktisk eller terapeutisk ståsted [Who gets to be a music student? Art didactic or therapeutic standpoint]. *Nordic Journal of Art & Research, 4*(2).

UN Committee on the Rights of Persons with Disabilities. (2016). *General Comment No. 4 (2016) on the Right to Inclusive Education.* Retrieved from https://www.ohchr.org/en/treaty-bodies/crpd

UNESCO & United Nations Children's Fund. (2024). *Global report on early childhood care and education: The right to a strong foundation.* https://doi.org/10.54675/FWQA2113.

United Nations. (1989). *Convention on the rights of the child.* https://www.ohchr.org/en/instruments-mechanisms/instruments/convention-rights-child

United Nations Convention on the Rights of the Child [UNCRC]. (2013). General comments No. 17 on the right of the child to rest, leisure, play, recreational activities, cultural life, and the arts (ar. 31). In The convention on the rights of the child. (Issue 3).

Utdanningsdirektoratet. (2017). *Læreplan.* Utdanningsdirektoratet. https://www.udir.no

Vatnedalen Vik, A. L., Thiedemann, M., & Brennskag Nettum, L. (2023). Synd med beina, dans med øynene—sangens muligheter li å inkludere alle. In A. H. Balsnes, L. A. Hagen, & S. Haukenes (Eds.), *Sangglede og stemmebruk i barnehagen* (pp. 135–148).

Wölfl, A. (2014). *Gewaltprävention mit Musik: Empirische Wirkungsanalyse eines musiktherapeutischen Projektmodells.* Reichert.

CHAPTER 6

Music Therapy in Mental Health and Well-being

Relevant articles for music therapy in mental health and well-being (United Nations, 1989).

Article 12—Respect for the views of the child

Children have the right to express their views freely in all matters affecting them, with those views being given due weight according to their age and maturity.

Article 13—Freedom of expression

Children have the right to seek, receive, and impart information and ideas of all kinds, including through artistic expression.

Article 24—Health and health services

Children have the right to the highest attainable standard of health, including mental health services.

Article 27—Adequate standard of living

Children have the right to a standard of living adequate for their physical, mental, spiritual, moral, and social development.

(*continued*)

V. Krüger, K. M. Murphy, *Child-Centred Music Therapy*,
https://doi.org/10.1007/978-3-031-85724-9_6

(continued)
Article 29—Education: Aims of education

This article promotes the development of the child's personality, talents, and mental and physical abilities to their fullest potential.

Right to Play, Leisure, and Culture (Article 31): This article guarantees children's right to engage in play and recreational activities appropriate to their age, as well as to participate freely in cultural life and the arts.

Introduction

In this chapter we review literature on music therapy as it relates to the mental health and well-being of children. Mental health as it relates to children is not the absence of a diagnosed mental disorder, rather it includes "reaching developmental and emotional milestones, learning healthy socials skill and how to cope when problems arise" (Center for Disease Control [CDC], 2024a, sec.2, para. 1). There are several factors that will influence children's mental health including genetic and biological factors (Hoy et al., 2023), unstable and unsafe environments, and adverse childhood experiences (ACEs). ACEs are traumatic events that occur when a child is between the ages of 0 and 17 and may include experiencing or witnessing violence, abuse or neglect, having a family member who is diagnosed with a mental disorder or died by suicide, or instability in living condition due to parental separation or incarceration (CDC, 2024b)

The WHO (2024) reports that one in seven children aged 10–19 have experienced a mental disorder, with depression, anxiety, and behavioural disorders being most common. Further, the WHO notes that suicide is the leading cause of death among 15- to 29-year-olds. It is important to remember that children who are not diagnosed with a mental health condition may experience challenges to their overall well-being that may negatively impact their ability to cope with everyday stressors. Symptoms that may be indicative of a mental health issue can appear anytime during childhood/adolescence and often change over time. Early diagnosis and treatment are essential as mental health conditions can interfere with healthy development (CDC, 2024a). This recommendation is consistent with

Article 24 of the UNCRC (1989), yet mental health disorders in children and adolescents often go undertreated (Radez et al., 2021).

Children and adolescents may receive treatment for mental health issues in a variety of settings including schools, outpatient clinics, in-patient facilities, residential programmes, juvenile detention centres (Mojtabai & Olfson, 2024) or community health settings (Thomson et al., 2023). Treatment goals typically focus on emotional regulation, coping skills, stress management and strengthening social support (Bauer et al., 2021). This work focuses on enhancing the ability to regulate emotions, manage stress, and engage in relationships. Additionally, it promotes sound decision-making processes and adaptive coping mechanisms in response to life's challenges. By addressing these areas, mental health interventions aim to foster resilience and well-being, potentially mitigating the onset of more severe mental health issues. Early and sustained support in these areas not only improves emotional and social functioning but also contributes to better academic outcomes and long-term life satisfaction (Kaku et al., 2022).

There are a myriad of contemporary psychotherapy approaches/orientations when working with children and adolescents including brief solution-focused therapies, cognitive behavioural therapy, play therapy, and family therapy (Cook-Cottone et al., 2019). Music therapists may incorporate strategies and techniques from these approaches into their clinical work; they may work from a music-centred orientation (Aigen, 2005) or adapt methods from other music therapy models such as Nordoff-Robbins (Pèrez-Eizaguirre et al., 2022), Bonny Method of Guided Imagery and Music (Band, 2019), and Analytical Music Therapy (Strehlow, 2009). This wide range of treatment approaches that music therapists can choose from allow flexibility and a collaborative approach to in the provision of music therapy.

Mental health challenges among children and adolescents can encompass a wide spectrum of issues, including anxiety, depression, and behavioural disorders, all of which can have profound impacts on their development and daily functioning (Salari et al., 2024). The treatment approaches for these challenges often vary depending on the severity of the condition. Inpatient care, which involves staying at a hospital or specialized facility, is generally reserved for more severe cases that require intensive monitoring and support. In contrast, outpatient care allows the child or adolescent to remain at home while attending regular therapy or counselling sessions, addressing less severe issues or serving as a transitional step from inpatient treatment. Both inpatient and outpatient interventions share the goal of improving the young person's mental health by helping them build coping mechanisms and resilience for healthier long-term outcomes (Kaku et al., 2022). Inpatient and outpatient care are often integrated to provide a comprehensive approach to treating children and adolescents with mental health issues. Initially, inpatient care offers intensive support and monitoring for severe conditions, allowing for thorough assessments and stabilization through medication management, therapy, and skills training.

Despite music therapy being a common component of mental health treatment for children and adolescents, empirical evidence supporting its effectiveness is limited. Recent meta-analyses suggest that music therapy can significantly reduce depression (Gold et al., 2004) internalizing symptoms (e.g. depression and anxiety) (Geipel et al., 2018) and aggressive behaviour (Ye et al., 2021) among children and adolescents. Authors from these meta-analyses note that while the results are promising, more research is needed. Research, both quantitative and qualitative, related to group music to treat mental health disorders in children and adolescents is increasing with representation from six of the seven continents of the world: Asia (e.g. Yun & Chung; 2019), Australia (e.g. Hense & McFerran, 2017), Africa (e.g. dos Santos, 2019), Europe (e.g. Pèrez-Eizaguirre et al., 2022), North America (Shuman et al., 2016), and South America (e.g. Albornoz, 2011).

Inpatient and Outpatient Mental Health

Group Dynamics and Interpersonal Relationships: The role of the music therapist is to facilitate emotional expression, relaxation, and social connections among participants. Music therapy creates safe spaces for exploring complex emotions, fostering trust and validation among peers.

Fun as a Therapeutic Element: The concept of "fun" plays a critical role in engaging children and adolescents in music therapy, supporting emotional expression and therapeutic progress.

(*continued*)

(continued)

Development of Therapeutic Programmes: Tailored music therapy programmes address specific needs of populations, such as paediatric patients awaiting mental health services or adolescents in psychiatric settings. Programmes are designed to overcome challenges inherent in these transitional phases.

Community and Participatory Approaches: Community music therapy emphasizes participation and collective experiences, enhancing self-efficacy, confidence, and social skills among young people.

Culturally Relevant Frameworks: Integrating indigenous health models and practices into music therapy can enhance therapeutic outcomes, emphasizing holistic approaches to well-being. Culturally sensitive practices recognize the diverse backgrounds and experiences of participants.

Challenging Norms and Marginalization: Music therapists play a role in reframing societal discourses around gender, sexuality, and other identities, promoting equity and inclusivity in therapeutic practice.

Promotion of Emotional Skills: Music therapy can effectively develop emotional skills in adolescents with mental health conditions, employing a combination of music-based and non-music-based methods.

Addressing Trauma and PTSD: Interactive audio-visual therapy shows promise in alleviating PTSD symptoms in adolescents, particularly in trauma-affected populations.

Music Therapy in Inpatient Mental Health Care

Inpatient care, which involves staying at a hospital or specialized facility, is generally reserved for more severe cases that require intensive monitoring and support or medication management. Music therapy is often integrated into inpatient therapeutic programmes that may include other psychotherapeutic modalities and psychopharmacology. In this setting music therapists often address goals related to self-expression, improving self-esteem, increasing positive socialization, and increasing knowledge and use of coping skills (Johnson & Heiderscheit, 2018). Other goal areas reported in the literature include validation of feelings, increasing group cohesion, frustration tolerance, and self-awareness (e.g. Rosado, 2019). Music therapists use a variety of music therapy methods including song discussion, song writing, improvisation, music listening, music games, and re-creation to address clinical goals (e.g. Johnson & Heiderscheit, 2018; Rosado, 2019).

There is limited body research on the efficacy of music therapy on inpatient mental health units for children and adolescents. Most of this research employed qualitative methodology to gain an understanding of how children/adolescents view their experiences in music therapy. It is important to highlight that in all the following studies the child/adolescent's voice held the privileged position in the interviews, rather than that of the music therapist or other members of the interdisciplinary team.

Rosado (2019) interviewed 14 adolescents on an inpatient crisis stabilization unit about their experiences in group music therapy. Results indicated that participation in group music therapy affirmed participants' strengths and coping resources, integrated cognitive and affective processes and provided continuity of experiences (p. 133). Respondents also noted the importance of connecting with peers and experiencing others' emotions in sessions helped them to develop empathy. The participants noted that music was part of their life before being hospitalized, they were able to bring their musical identity into the hospital helping them to feel more comfortable.

Utilizing a multiple case study design, including semi-structured interviews and participant observations, Klyve and Rolvsjord (2023) explored the nuanced ways children engage with music therapy in a Norwegian hospital setting. In the study the researchers sought to capture the children's personal experiences and perspectives. The concept of "fun" emerged as a central theme, reflecting its multifaceted role in therapy. Far from being merely an element of enjoyment, "fun" was found to encapsulate deeper, existential aspects of the therapeutic process, revealing its significance in fostering engagement, emotional expression, and therapeutic progress. The narrative approach employed allowed for a rich exploration of the children's experiences, demonstrating that "fun" in music therapy serves as a vital component in addressing their complex mental health needs, offering both a source of relief and a meaningful therapeutic tool.

The following case vignette is an excerpt from Klyve and Rolvsjord (2023) which highlights children's diverse ways of expressing themselves while engaging in music experiences.

Kristin Kristin calls out into the microphone when she arrives at the music room, "Hello! Hello!". The sound lingers for a while, then it becomes silent. "Whoa, there are two microphones!" she suddenly shouts, discovering an additional microphone in the room. "Yes", I say, sitting down. "Why?" Kristin asks. I suggest it might be because someone else has been in the room. But Kristin is of another opinion, suggesting that it is because she is supposed to sit one way with one of the microphones, and I with the other one, and then she sits down with her back to me. I ask if Kristin remembers anything of what she and I have done together in the music therapy sessions. "Mmm", Kristin says cautiously. Then there is a long moment of silence between us. "We have played music", Kristin says. "Yes", I answer, following up asking her if she has played any instruments. Kristin responds with a quick and clear "yes". "Yes, we have. And we have also played a particular song quite a bit, haven't we?" I ask. Kristin gets up, heading for the computer. She clicks and writes a while before she finds a song from a film from which we have played many songs together. Kristin puts on the song and we watch the music video together. "I wonder how do you think it was to play instruments and sing while you were here at the unit?" Kristin continues clicking and writing on the computer. It's quiet again. "Fun" Kristin says after a little while. I point at the crayons, and say that Kristin may draw, if she wants to. Kristin says, "Yes", and starts to draw immediately. She is concentrated on drawing for a long time. I occasionally ask some questions, but it is completely silent while she draws. She sometimes goes back and forth to the computer where the photo of a girl from the music video is displayed. The girl is the one who sings the song that Kristin and I have played a lot together during the sessions (Klyve & Rolvsjord, 2023).

Music Therapy in Outpatient Mental Health Settings

Outpatient care and community programmes (1) allow children and adolescents to remain at home while attending regular therapy or counselling sessions, (2) address less severe issues, or (3) serve as a transitional step from inpatient treatment. As with inpatient treatment, outpatient programmes share the goal of improving the young person's mental health by helping them build coping mechanisms and resilience for healthier long-term outcomes (Kaku et al., 2022). Inpatient and outpatient care are often integrated to provide a comprehensive approach to treating children and adolescents with mental health issues. Initially, inpatient care offers intensive support and monitoring for severe conditions, allowing for thorough assessments and stabilization through medication management, therapy, and skills training.

Research related to music therapy in outpatient mental health treatment facilities and community-based programmes for children and adolescents is also limited with promising results. Results from quantitative and qualitative studies set the foundation for inclusion of music therapy in these treatment programmes as well as the need for continued research.

Gold et al. (2017) investigated changes over time in children and adolescents who received music therapy in outpatient or special education centres in Vienna. Participants received individual music therapy sessions primarily involving clinical improvisation, along with other active and receptive music therapy methods. Results indicated participation may have improved participant quality of life, based on both child and parent report.

The efficacy of multimodal music therapy (MMT) (a combination of music therapy and cognitive behavioural therapy) was compared to treatment as usual for children ages 8–12 with anxiety disorders receiving therapy in an outpatient clinic in Ulm, Germany (Goldbeck & Ellerkamp, 2012). Participants received three individual and nine group sessions. Music therapy methods used were selected from the treatment manual by the therapists, not the children. Results indicated that children receiving MMT reported a significant decrease in anxiety as compared to those in the control group immediately following the treatment. They remained significantly lower four months post study completion.

Shuman et al. (2016) conducted a retrospective mixed method study to evaluate the impact of group music therapy on the mood states of adolescent inpatients and outpatients at a psychiatric hospital. The study involved

352 predominantly white, non-Hispanic patients aged 12–21, who completed 596 mood assessments using the Fast Assessment of Children's Emotions (FACE) before and after music therapy sessions. The results revealed a high probability of positive mood changes following the sessions, indicating a significant immediate impact on the participants' mood states. This research provides preliminary evidence that group music therapy offered as part of the treatment in both inpatient and outpatient settings can positively affect the mood of adolescent patients with psychiatric disorders.

Hense and McFerran (2017) investigated the underexplored area of musical identity focusing on young people with mental illness and subsequent recovery. The researchers conducted and analysed in-depth interviews with participants in a music therapy programme at a youth mental health service in Australia. The findings illustrate how aspects of the participants' pathology manifested as musical symptoms during acute illness and how these young individuals actively engaged in processes to reconstruct and express their musical identities within their communities. The study emphasizes the critical role of music therapy in aiding recovery and advocates for the integration of community-based music services to support young people in their mental health journeys.

Community-Based Music Therapy Programmes

Community-based music programmes have been developed to address the mental health needs of adolescents. As an example, Baker et al. (2018) explored the impact of contextual factors on the well-being outcomes of young people participating in an artist-led group songwriting programme. The study observed participants in a two-day songwriting workshop. They analysed video footage, field notes, and artefacts to identify the effect of the programme on the well-being of participants. They identified three key themes during their data analysis that contributed to well-being: creating a sense of safety, fostering fun, and encouraging young people to push beyond their boundaries. Sub-themes such as honest feedback, high-energy rituals, and a focus on artistic excellence were crucial in shaping these outcomes. The findings highlight how the songwriting environment can be tailored to support the well-being of young participants, offering valuable insights for music therapy and other fields that employ group songwriting to enhance youth well-being. They also support the notion of "fun" as identified by Klyve and Rolvsjord (2023).

Mitchell (2019, 2021) describes the *Coffee House*, a biannual musical performance event at an adolescent mental health treatment facility in Southwestern Ontario, Canada. The event, open to all clients and staff, is organized by the facility's music therapist and serves as an example of community music therapy. This programme demonstrates how participatory settings can offer a new and distinct experience compared to traditional presentational performance settings. Mitchell (2021) interviewed adolescents who performed in the *Coffee House*. Results of her interviews suggest that the adolescent performers experienced an "expansion of their overall self-identities" (p. 39) which included new beliefs about their musical performance abilities. This led to an improved self-concept and self-identity (Mitchell, 2021).

Music Therapy with Children Who Have Experienced Sexual Abuse and Exploitation

Children and adolescents who have experienced sexual abuse and exploitation are at heightened risk for adverse outcomes related to mental and physical health (Hailes et al., 2019). Children and adolescents who have faced sexual abuse and exploitation often carry deep psychological scars that can manifest as anxiety, depression, post-traumatic stress disorder (PTSD), and difficulties in trusting others (Massullo et al., 2023). Traditional talk therapy may be challenging for these children and adolescents, as verbalizing traumatic experiences can be overwhelming. Additionally, as noted by Lefevre (2004), they may lack the cognitive and language necessary to benefit from traditional verbal therapy. Music therapy, however, provides a non-verbal and creative outlet for expression, making it a powerful treatment modality for processing trauma. It has the potential to offer a unique and sensitive way to address trauma, support recovery, and foster resilience.

Suzuki et al. (2023) conducted a systematic review of current research on music therapy for adolescent survivors of sexual abuse. Their goal was to enhance understanding of its application by identifying primary studies that focus on the context of care, participant age, therapy duration, therapist qualifications, clinical objectives, methodologies, and the associated benefits and challenges during adolescence. Clinical goals and outcomes identified included development of social skills, emotional regulation, and expression of feelings. The authors indicated participation in music therapy promoted positive affective experiences, helped in the communication of ideas and feelings, and in the building or reconstruction of identity. Additionally, participation in music therapy was found empowered survivors to explore their identities and regain self-worth through creative expression, emphasizing positive reinforcement and celebrating small achievements to boost confidence and resilience.

Strehlow (2009) describes the use of analytical music therapy in her work with children who have been sexually abused. Analytical music therapy is defined as the analytically informed symbolic use of improvised music by the music therapist and client. "It is used as a creative tool with which to explore the client's inner life to provide the way forward for growth and greater self-knowledge" (Priestley, 1994, p. 3). Key concepts include the importance of the client–therapist relationship, which, in theory, will allow for the creation of a safe environment. Free improvisation, composed music, and singing songs are used to help children demonstrate how they interact with others, share their story, integrate the experience, and develop resources to cope with memories of past abuse. Strehlow also identifies several key functions of music in the therapy process: (1) music creates distance (p. 174), (2) music provides a space for good experiences (p. 175), (3) music makes strong emotions such as fear audible (p. 176), and (4) music puts the emphasis on emotional experience (p. 177).

Schrader and Wendland (2012) describe the process they followed in the development of a music therapy programme for child survivors of sexual exploitation and violence in Cambodia. The authors incorporated a variety of music therapy methods to support programming that was already in place in the Life Skills class and weekly music groups. Music therapy methods included singing, song discussion, song writing, music-assisted relaxation, instrument play and improvisation and movement. Songwriting was used to help the girls remember their rights as children. This experience reinforced the rights enshrined in the UNCRC (1989), specifically the right to safety, education, and health care. Other methods were used to address goals related to emotional expression, coping skills, minimizing isolation, social skill development.

Article 12 of UNCRC (1989) reminds us that children have the right to be active decision-makers in their treatment. Christenbury (2017) offers an example of a collaborative approach when working with children who have been physically and sexually abused. She noticed her client (referred to as Leah) had shown an interest in using stories, art, and music as vehicles for creative and emotional self-expression. Based on these observations, Christenbury proposed that Leah and she would work together to create a book related to the feelings of happiness, sadness, and anger. Leah would draw a pictorial representation of the feeling, and Christenbury would write a song based on the drawing. The completed project resulted in a book, and accompanying CD which included recordings of the songs that Christenbury wrote. Again, in line with Article 12, Christenbury encouraged Leah to have "a voice and sense of control" in the sessions (p. 7). Leah often refused to listen to the therapist composed songs, and Christenbury honoured that request. Additionally, Christenbury allowed Leah the time needed to express the emotions she selected to represent in the book.

Minor Migrants

Ali 18 years old and has a multicultural background. He has lived in Norway for about three years, most of the time in various institutions. As a 15-year-old boy, he fled to Norway from his home country as a refugee. He travelled alone and during his journey he experienced many dangerous and unpleasant situations. During the working phase of music therapy, Ali brought lyrics to the session. Through a collaborative process of trying and failing, Ali discovered a way he could sing the lyrics. First, he sang in his mother tongue, and later in Norwegian. Based on the collaborative process, recordings were made, and performances held. Ali used his songwriting to express his feelings and thoughts. He wrote at home and brought lyrics to the music sessions. We used our time to look at grammar and fix language errors. He worked with lyrics for months before Ali was satisfied. He used songwriting as a form of a diary account, but he also had ambitions of being a songwriter and performer. Both of the goals were taken into consideration. Ali told the music therapist that it was easier for him to express himself through a song than through a conversation and that writing songs helped him to articulate thoughts that otherwise would be difficult to communicate directly through conversation (Krüger et al., 2018).

Music therapy is an increasingly recognized intervention for supporting the mental health and well-being of minor migrants, including refugees, asylum seekers, and unaccompanied minors (Krüger & Diaz, 2023). Programmes are provided in educational and community settings to support children who face a range of challenges, including trauma, cultural dislocation, and difficulties in adjusting to new environments. Music therapy offers a unique and culturally adaptable approach to address these complex needs, providing a non-verbal, creative outlet that transcends language barriers and supports emotional recovery (Heynen et al., 2022).

Group music therapy fosters social cohesion among displaced children, helping them form friendships and regain normalcy (Baker & Jones, 2006). Additionally, music therapy serves as a shared activity for families, promoting emotional healing and strengthening bonds. Similarly, Weiss and Bensimon (2019) found that structured environments in group music therapy programmes were critical for establishing belonging and personal expression. A unique music therapy group programme was developed for pre-school children who were forced to evacuate from their homes in the Gaza Strip along with their families (Felsenstein, 2013). The group programme sought to build trust and group cohesion. A flexible session structure was followed each week. Music experiences were chosen to meet the needs expressed by the children in the opening song. Sessions ended with a closing song that summarized what occurred during the group. Music experiences were chosen based on their ability to foster group cooperation and foster a sense of belonging and containment among group members. This allowed group members "to hear and be heard" (p. 14). Felsentein also describes the music therapy methods or experiences that were not helpful. This serves as an important reminder of our ethical obligation to not cause harm.

Enge and Stige (2022) describe how the inclusion of music therapy in primary schools can support refugee children's readiness to collaborate with peers through interconnected emotional and social processes. Key elements of the programme include self-regulation, social negotiation, and building a shared musical repertoire, all of which reinforce each other. Emotional readiness, especially affect-regulation, is essential for effective social participation. By addressing both emotional and social needs, music therapy can play a crucial role in promoting refugee children's social well-being and development within the school setting.

Music programmes outside of traditional music therapy settings may also meet the needs of migrant or refugee children. Roaldsnes (2017) underscores the importance of music groups for unaccompanied minor refugees, emphasizing their role in fostering emotional change, coping strategies, and a sense of belonging. The study reveals that participation in music groups provided these young refugees with a safe space where they could express emotions, navigate their experiences, and connect with others. Through these musical interactions, participants not only experienced emotional relief but also developed supportive relationships that enhanced their sense of community. This social support was crucial for their well-being, helping them to feel more grounded and secure in their new environment. The findings suggest that music groups can play a significant role in promoting emotional resilience and social integration among unaccompanied minors, highlighting the therapeutic potential of communal music-making for vulnerable refugee populations.

Storsve, Westby, and Ruud (2010) examine the role of music in fostering hope among youth in a Palestinian refugee camp, emphasizing its psychosocial support in educational settings. Their work illustrates how music projects can enhance self-esteem and social recognition, serving as a bridge to connect individuals and promote resilience amid trauma and conflict. In sum, these studies underline the value of integrating music therapy into educational systems to support diverse student groups facing trauma and displacement.

Implementing music therapy or music programmes with migrants has challenges, including cultural sensitivity and the risk of re-traumatization. Edwards (2023) emphasizes the need for culturally informed practices to prevent harm in all music therapy settings. Comte (2016) reminds that while music therapy can effectively transcend cultural and language barriers, it may also unintentionally reinforce assumptions, such as viewing refugees as a homogenous group defined by trauma. To promote empowerment, therapists should challenge these narratives and be mindful of the influence of neo-colonial attitudes in their approaches and consider power dynamics inherent in music therapy practices (Comte, 2016). This is especially important considering GC. No 14 (UNCRC, 2013) which reminds music therapist we have to be aware and respectful of a child's cultural identity and work to create music experiences that uphold cultural beliefs and practice.

Music Therapy for Sex Offenders

For individuals who have committed sexual offences, traditional therapeutic methods often focus on cognitive-behavioural techniques, which aim to change distorted thinking patterns and prevent reoffending. Oosthuizen (2018) presents a compelling account of the Support Programme for Abuse Reactive Children (SPARC), a music therapy initiative in South Africa designed for young sex offenders. SPARC combines active music experiences (e.g. drumming, improvisation, and songwriting) with receptive experiences (e.g. music listening and imagery exploration). The programme aims to enhance self-esteem, facilitate emotional expression, provide personal insights, and develop healthy social skills by focusing on how musical experiences can help release intense emotions and explore social dynamics. As such, music therapy offers a non-verbal outlet for sex offenders, helping them navigate emotional regulation, impulsivity, and complex feelings associated with their actions. Through improvisation and songwriting, participants can articulate feelings that are difficult to express in traditional therapy, allowing them to confront unresolved issues like anger and guilt. Engaging with music enables offenders to learn emotional regulation skills, such as creating calming music to reduce anxiety or using active music-making to safely express frustration. Additionally, music therapy fosters empathy and perspective-taking by encouraging offenders to connect with the emotions of others, enhancing their understanding of the impact of their actions on victims. Group sessions promote social skills through collaborative music-making, while the non-confrontational nature of music therapy can reduce resistance to treatment. This approach allows for flexibility in addressing individual needs and preferences, increasing motivation and engagement.

Gaps in the Research

Identifying research gaps in the field of music therapy for children and adolescent mental health can help guide future studies and improve therapeutic outcomes. In reviewing the related research, it is evident that most of these studies involve research on children, rather than with children. This is an affront to Article 12 of the UNCRC (1989) which requires children to be active participants in their treatment. Klyve (2019) highlights the importance of listening to children's voices in research. Music therapists who work with children in mental health settings, clinically or as researchers, would do well to give Klyve's position careful consideration in their clinical work and research endeavours.

One notable gap is the limited exploration of how musical identity evolves during recovery from mental illness, as highlighted by Hense et al. (2015). More research is needed to understand how young individuals reconstruct and express their musical identities within their communities and how this process aids in their recovery. Additionally, while studies like those by Baker et al. (2018) emphasize the importance of contextual factors in group songwriting programmes, there is a need for more detailed investigations into how specific elements of the therapeutic environment contribute to well-being outcomes. The impact of group music therapy on mood states, as explored by Shuman et al. (2016), also warrants further research, particularly in diverse demographic settings to understand the broader applicability of these findings.

Additionally, there is a need for more longitudinal studies to assess the long-term benefits of music therapy, as current research often emphasizes short-term outcomes. The cultural and socioeconomic diversity of outpatient populations is another area that requires more attention, as most studies are conducted within specific cultural contexts, limiting the generalizability of findings. Understanding the underlying mechanisms of how music therapy facilitates emotional expression and stress reduction is also crucial, as this can inform more targeted and effective interventions.

Moreover, the role of community music therapy events, such as the Coffee House described by Mitchell (2019, 2021), in fostering self-efficacy and confidence through participatory settings, needs more empirical support to validate its effectiveness across different populations and settings. While qualitative research provides valuable insights into the experiences of individuals in music therapy, there is a need for more mixed-methods studies that combine qualitative and quantitative data to provide a comprehensive understanding of music therapy's impact on recovery. Addressing these gaps can provide a more nuanced understanding of how music therapy can support mental health recovery and help tailor interventions to meet the diverse needs of individuals in recovery. Lastly, the limited research on how music therapy affects family and social relationships suggests a gap in investigating the broader impact of music therapy on adolescents' family dynamics and peer relationships. Addressing these gaps can provide a more comprehensive understanding of music therapy's role in adolescent mental health and help tailor interventions to meet the diverse needs of this population.

Research gaps regarding music therapy for children and adolescents who have experienced sexual abuse and exploitation can be identified in several areas. While existing studies, such as the systematic review by Suzuki et al. (2023), provide insights into the therapeutic benefits and contexts of music therapy, further investigation is needed into the specific methodologies employed across diverse settings. Research exploring the variations in therapeutic approaches, such as different music therapy techniques (e.g. improvisation, songwriting, or active vs receptive methods), could illuminate which strategies are most effective for different symptoms and trauma histories. Another significant gap is the need for comprehensive studies exploring the integration of music therapy with other therapeutic modalities (e.g. cognitive-behavioural therapy or art therapy) to develop more holistic treatment frameworks. Finally, ethical considerations, including consent and the potential risks of re-traumatization, require further examination to establish best practices for safeguarding vulnerable populations in music therapy settings. By addressing these gaps, future research can enhance the understanding of music therapy's role in supporting recovery and resilience among children and adolescents who have experienced sexual abuse and exploitation.

The increasing recognition of music therapy as a valuable intervention for forcibly displaced minors in educational settings highlights several critical research gaps that warrant further exploration. First, longitudinal studies assessing the long-term effects of music therapy on mental health and well-being are needed to understand how these benefits evolve over time. Additionally, more research on culturally specific approaches is essential to ensure interventions are adaptable to the diverse ethnic backgrounds of minor migrants, promoting culturally informed practices and minimizing re-traumatization risks. Standardized metrics for measuring outcomes in music therapy are currently lacking, which hinders evidence-based practices. Moreover, the potential for technology, such as virtual music therapy, to broaden access to underserved populations remains underexplored. Research on integrating music therapy with other support services—psychological, educational, and social—could lead to more holistic frameworks for aiding these minors. Furthermore, investigating the neurobiological mechanisms behind the therapeutic benefits of music therapy for trauma recovery can enhance theoretical understanding. Comparative studies assessing the effectiveness of music therapy against other therapeutic modalities would also be beneficial. While the benefits of group dynamics in music therapy are noted, further research is necessary to understand the specific interactions that foster community building and emotional healing. Lastly, insights from music therapists working with these populations can inform training and support systems to improve service delivery. More research is needed to compare different therapeutic modalities (such as drumming and songwriting) in their effectiveness for various offender types, as well as to investigate the underlying mechanisms that facilitate emotional expression and social skills development.

Recommendations for Practice

The implications for practice based on meta-analyses and various studies underscore the significant potential of music therapy in reducing symptoms such as depression, anxiety, distress, and emotional dysregulation, particularly in group settings. Research by Gold et al. (2004) and Geipel et al. (2018) confirms measurable improvements, especially in behavioural and developmental disorders. Individual treatments, while less studied, also show improved outcomes, as seen in trials by Porter et al. (2017) and McFerran et al. (2018). To enhance the effectiveness of music therapy, practitioners should consider the three elements of evidence-based practice: the best available research, practice wisdom, and the needs, values and preferences of the child.

In addition to the traditional music therapy methods and their variations, interactive audio-visual methods are innovative approaches to addressing PTSD among children (Christenbury, 2017) and adolescents (Iyendo et al., 2024). Clinicians are encouraged to utilize technology as a means of creating immersive experiences that combine music, visuals, and storytelling to engage clients more deeply in their therapeutic processes. Regardless of the methods used, facilitators must also pay close attention to group dynamics, ensuring that each member feels heard and supported. Regular check-ins and feedback sessions can help assess individual needs and adapt the therapy accordingly (Preyde et al., 2015).

Moreover, incorporating elements of fun and engagement is crucial, especially for children. Practitioners should consider hands-on activities like music games or collaborative songwriting, which can enhance enjoyment and participation. Klyve and Rolvsjord (2023) highlight the importance of fun in therapeutic processes for children. Community-based programmes, like Mitchell's (2019, 2021) *Coffee House* event, demonstrate the value of participatory music therapy settings in fostering self-efficacy and social connection. Practitioners can organize similar events that encourage families and community members to engage in music-making together, strengthening bonds and promoting a supportive environment.

Finally, training caregivers in music therapy techniques can further assist them in supporting children through trauma processing, as described by Colegrove et al. (2018). Workshops for caregivers that provide practical strategies, such as using music for calming or emotional expression, can empower them to integrate music therapy into everyday interactions with children. Collectively, these hands-on suggestions highlight the versatility of music therapy across cultural contexts and the importance of integrating it into various clinical and community settings to enhance emotional and psychological well-being.

References

Aigen, K. (2005). *Music-centered music therapy*. Barcelona Publishers.

Albornoz, Y. (2011). The effects of group improvisational music therapy on depression in young people and adults with substance abuse: A randomized controlled trial. *Nordic Journal of Music Therapy, 20*(3), 208–224. https://doi.org/10.1080/08098131.2010.522717

Baker, F., & Jones, C. (2006). The effect of music therapy services on classroom behaviours of newly arrived refugee students in Australia: A pilot study. *Emotional and Behavioural Difficulties, 11*(4), 249–260. https://doi.org/10.1080/13632750601022170

Baker, F. A., Jeanneret, N., & Clarkson, A. (2018). Contextual factors and wellbeing outcomes: Ethnographic analysis of an artist-led group songwriting program with young people. *Psychology of Music, 46*(2), 266–280. https://doi.org/10.1177/0305735617709520

Band, J. P. (2019). Guided imagery and music with children and young people. In D. E. Grocke (Ed.), *Guided imagery and music: The Bonny method and beyond* (pp. 79–96). Barcelona Publishers.

Bauer, A., Stevens, M., Purtscheller, D., Knapp, M., Fonagy, P., Evans-Lacko, S., & Paul, J. (2021). Mobilising social support to improve mental health for children and adolescents: A systematic review using principles of realist synthesis. *PLoS One, 16*(5), e0251750. https://doi.org/10.1371/journal.pone.0251750

Center for Disease Control and Prevention (CDC). (2024a, August 20). *About children's mental health*. https://www.c.gov/children-mental-health/about/index.html

Center for Disease Control and Prevention (CDC). (2024b, October 8). *About adverse childhood experiences*. https://www.cdc.gov/aces/about/

Christenbury, K. R. (2017). I will follow you: The combined use of songwriting and art to promote healing in a child who has been traumatized. *Music Therapy Perspectives, 35*(1), 1–12. https://doi.org/10.1093/mtp/miv005

Colegrove, V., Havighurst, S. S., Kehoe, C. E., & Jacobsen, S. L. (2018). Pilot randomized controlled trial of tuning relationships with music: Intervention for parents with a trauma history and their adolescents. *Child Abuse & Neglect, 79*, 259–268. https://doi.org/10.1016/j.chiabu.2018.01.001

Comte, R. (2016). Neo-colonialism in music therapy: A critical interpretive synthesis of the literature concerning music therapy practice with refugees. *Voices: A World Forum for Music Therapy, 16*(3). https://doi.org/10.15845/voices.v16i3.865

Cook-Cottone, C. P., Kane, L., & Anderson, L. (2019). *The elements of counseling children and adolescents*. Springer Publishing Company.

Edwards, J. (2023). Cultural humility in music therapy practice. In L. E. Beer & J. C. Birnbaum (Eds.), *Trauma-informed music therapy* (pp. 28–36). Routledge.

Enge, K. E. A., & Stige, B. (2022). Musical pathways to the peer community: A collective case study of refugee children's use of music therapy. *Nordic Journal of Music Therapy, 31*(1), 7–24. https://doi.org/10.1080/08098131.2021.1891130

Felsenstein, R. (2013). From uprooting to replanting: On post-trauma group music therapy for pre-school children. *Nordic Journal of Music Therapy, 22*(1), 69–85. https://doi.org/10.1080/08098131.2012.667824

Geipel, J., Koenigb, J., Hillecke, T. K., Reschch, F., & Kaess, M. (2018). Music-based interventions to reduce internalizing symptoms in children and adolescents: A meta-analysis. *Journal of Affective Disorders, 225*, 647–656.

Gold, C., Voracek, M., & Wigram, T. (2004). Effects of music therapy for children and adolescents with psychopathology: A meta-analysis. *Journal of Child Psychology and Psychiatry, 45*(6), 1054–1059.

Gold, C., Saarikallio, S., Crooke, A. H. D., & McFerran, K. S. (2017). Group music therapy as a preventive intervention for young people at risk: A cluster-randomized trial. *Journal of Music Therapy, 54*(2), 133–160.

Goldbeck, L., & Ellerkamp, T. (2012). A randomized controlled trial of multimodal music therapy for children with anxiety disorders. *Journal of Music Therapy, 49*(4), 395–413.

Hailes, H. P., Yu, R., Danese, A., & Fazel, S. (2019). Long-term outcomes of childhood sexual abuse: An umbrella review. *The Lancet Psychiatry, 6*(10), 830–839. https://doi.org/10.1016/S2215-0366(19)30286-X

Hense, C., & McFerran, K. S. (2017). Promoting young people's musical identities to facilitate recovery from mental illness. *Journal of Youth Studies, 20*(8), 997–1012. https://doi.org/10.1080/13676261.2017.1287882

Hense, C., McFerran, K. S., Killackey, E., & McGorry, P. D. (2015). How can research practice promote young people's recovery from mental illness: A critical look at the Australian context. *Youth Voice Journal.* https://doi.org/10.1093/mtp/miz014

Heynen, E., Bruls, V., van Goor, S., Pat-El, R., Schoot, T., & van Hooren, S. (2022). A music therapy intervention for refugee children and adolescents in schools: A process evaluation using a mixed method design. *Children, 9*(10), 1434. https://doi.org/10.3390/children9101434

Hoy, N., Lynch, S. J., Waszczuk, M. A., Reppermund, S., & Mewton, L. (2023). Transdiagnostic biomarkers of mental illness across the lifespan: A systematic review examining the genetic and neural correlates of latent transdiagnostic dimensions of psychopathology in the general population. *Neuroscience and Biobehavioral Reviews, 155*, 105431. https://doi.org/10.1016/j.neubiorev.2023.105431

Iyendo, T. O., Makanjuola, O. B., & Ojo, T. M. (2024). Effect of audio-visual-based art and music therapy in reducing adolescents' post-traumatic stress disorder. *Journal of Adolescent Health, 74*(2), 283–291. https://doi.org/10.1016/j.jadohealth.2023.07.008

Johnson, K., & Heiderscheit, A. (2018). A survey of music therapy methods on adolescent inpatient mental health units. *Journal of Music Therapy, 55*(4), 463–488. https://doi.org/10.1093/jmt/thy015

Kaku, S. M., Sibeoni, J., Basheer, S., et al. (2022). Global child and adolescent mental health perspectives: Bringing change locally, while thinking globally. *Child and Adolescent Psychiatry and Mental Health, 16*(82). https://doi.org/10.1186/s13034-022-00512-8

Klyve, G. P. (2019). Whose knowledge? Epistemic injustice and challenges in hearing children's voices. *Voices: A World Forum for Music Therapy, 19*(3).

Klyve, G. P., & Rolvsjord, R. (2023). Moments of fun: Narratives of children's experiences of music therapy in mental health care. *Nordic Journal of Music Therapy, 32*(2), 100–120. https://doi.org/10.1080/08098131.2022.2055114

Krüger, V., & Diaz, E. (2023). The potential to meet the needs of refugees and other migrants through music therapy. *The Lancet Regional Health, 29, Article 100637*. https://doi.org/10.1016/j.lancha.2023.100637

Krüger, V., Nordanger, D. Ø., & Stige. (2018). Music therapy: Building bridges between a participatory approach and trauma-informed care in a child welfare setting. *Voices: A World Forum for Music Therapy, 18*(4) https://voices.no/index.php/voices/article/view/2593

Lefevre, M. (2004). Finding the key: Containing and processing traumatic sexual abuse. *The Arts in Psychotherapy, 31*(3), 137–152. https://doi.org/10.1016/j.aip.2004.05.001

Massullo, C., De Rossi, E., Carbone, G. A., Imperatori, C., Ardito, R. B., Adenzato, M., & Farina, B. (2023). Child maltreatment, abuse, and neglect: An umbrella review of their prevalence and definitions. *Clinical Neuropsychiatry, 20*(2), 72–99. https://doi.org/10.36131/cnfioritieditore20230201

McFerran, K. S., Hense, C., Koike, A., & Rickwood, D. (2018). Intentional music use to reduce psychological distress in adolescents accessing primary mental health care. *Clinical Child Psychology and Psychiatry, 23*(4), 567–581. https://doi.org/10.1177/1359104518767231

Mitchell, E. (2019). Community music therapy and participatory performance: Case study of a coffee house. *Voices: A World Forum for Music Therapy, 19*(1). https://doi.org/10.15845/voices.v19i1.2701

Mitchell, E. (2021). Performing identities and performing relationships: Community music therapy and adolescent mental health. *Music Therapy Perspectives, 39*(2), 195–203. https://doi.org/10.1093/mtp/miab004

Mojtabai, R., & Olfson, M. (2024). Trends in mental disorders in children and adolescents receiving treatment in the state mental health system. *Journal of the American Academy of Child & Adolescent Psychiatry*, PMID 39214290. https://doi.org/10.1016/j.jaac.2024.08.008

Oosthuizen, H. B. (2018). Working with and within chaos: The development of a music therapy program for young sex offenders in South Africa. *Voices: A World Forum for Music Therapy, 18*(4). https://doi.org/10.15845/voices.v18i4.2588

Pèrez-Eizaguirre, M., Dorado, A., Rodríguez-Brioso, M., & Privado, J. (2022). Efficacy of music therapy in the treatment of anxiety among children at social risk and those have committed child to parent violence. *Psychology of Music, 50*(1), 328–342.

Porter, S., McConnell, T., McLaughlin, K., Lynn, F., Cardwell, C., Braiden, H. J., Boylan, J., & Holmes, V. (2017). Music therapy for children and adolescents with behavioural and emotional problems: A randomised controlled trial. *The Journal of Child Psychology and Psychiatry, 58*(5), 586–594.

Preyde, M., Berends, A., Parekh, S., & Heintzman, J. (2015). Adolescents' evaluation of music therapy in an inpatient psychiatric unit: A quality improvement project. *Music Therapy Perspectives, 35*(1), 58–62. https://doi.org/10.1093/mtp/miv027

Priestley, M. (1994). *Essays on analytical music therapy*. Barcelona Publishers.

Radez, J., Reardon, T., Creswell, C., Lawrence, P. J., Evdoka-Burton, G., & Waite, P. (2021). Why do children and adolescents (not) seek and access professional help for their mental health problems? A systematic review of quantitative and qualitative studies. *European Child & Adolescent Psychiatry, 30*(2), 183–211. https://doi.org/10.1007/s00787-019-01469-4

Roaldsnes, M. H. (2017). *Musikk i helsefremmande arbeid med einslege mindreårige flyktningar. Ein kvalitativ studie av ei musikkgruppe for ungdom med bakgrunn som einslege flyktningbarn* [Music in health promoting work with unaccompanied minor refugees. A qualitative study of a music group for adolescents with a background as unaccompanied minor refugees] (Doctoral dissertation). Norwegian Academy of Music. https://brage.bibsys.no/xmlui/bitstream/handle/11250/2469525/RoaldsneAvhandling_nett.pdf

Rosado, A. (2019). Adolescents' experiences of music therapy on an inpatient crisis stabilization unit. *Music Therapy Perspectives, 37*(2), 133–140. https://doi.org/10.1093/mtp/miz004

Ruud, E. (2010). *Music therapy: A perspective from the humanities*. Barcelona Publishers.

Salari, N., Heidarian, P., Hassanabadi, M., et al. (2024). Global prevalence of social anxiety disorder in children, adolescents and youth: A systematic review and meta-analysis. *Journal of Prevention*. https://doi.org/10.1007/s10935-024-00789-9

dos Santos, A. (2019). Empathy and aggression in group music therapy with teenagers: A descriptive phenomenological study. *Music Therapy Perspectives, 37*(1), 14–27. https://doi.org/10.1093/mtp/miy024

Schrader, E. M., & Wendland, J. M. (2012). Music therapy programming at an aftercare center in Cambodia for survivors of child sexual exploitation and rape and their caregivers. *Social Work & Christianity, 39*(4), 390–406.

Shuman, J., Kennedy, H., DeWitt, P., Edelblute, A., & Wamboldt, M. Z. (2016). Group music therapy impacts mood states of adolescents in a psychiatric hospital setting. *The Arts in Psychotherapy, 49*, 50–56. https://doi.org/10.1016/j.aip.2016.03.001

Strehlow, G. (2009). The use of music therapy in treating sexually abused children. *Nordic Journal of Music Therapy, 18*(2), 167–183. https://doi.org/10.1080/08098130903062397

Suzuki, D. C., Monge, A., Silva, B. S., Viana, J. A., Suzuki, P. R., Annunciato Neto, R., & Vitalle, M. S. (2023). *Adolescent victims of sexual abuse and music therapy: A systematic review*. Research, Society and Development.

Thomson, A., Hariss, E., Peters-Corbett, A., Koppel, K., & Creswell, C. (2023). Barriers and facilitators of community-based implementation of evidence-based interventions in the UK, for children and young people's mental health promotion, prevention and treatment: Rapid scoping review. *BJPsych Open, 9*, e132, 1–8. https://doi.org/10.1192/bjo.2023.531

UN Committee on the Rights of the Child (UNCRC). (2013). *General comment No. 14 on the right of the child to have his or her best interests taken as a primary consideration (art. 3, para. 1)*. CRC/C/GC/14. Retrieved from https://www2.ohchr.org/english/bodies/crc/docs/gc/crc_c_gc_14_eng.pdf

United Nations. (1989). *Convention on the rights of the child*. https://www.ohchr.org/en/instruments-mechanisms/instruments/convention-rights-child

Weiss, C., & Bensimon, M. (2019). Group music therapy with uprooted teenagers: The importance of structure. *Nordic Journal of Music Therapy, 29*(1), 20–35. https://doi.org/10.1080/08098131.2019.1695281

World Health Organization (WHO). (2024, October 10). *Mental health of adolescents*. https://www.who.int/news-room/fact-sheets/detail/adolescent-mental-health

Ye, P., Huang, Z., Zhou, H., & Tang, Q. (2021). Music-based intervention to reduce aggressive behavior in children and adolescents: A meta-analysis. *Medicine, 100*(4), e23894. https://doi.org/10.1097/MD.0000000000023894

CHAPTER 7

Music Therapy in Paediatric Care for Children, Adolescents, and Their Families

Introduction

Relevant articles of the Convention on the Rights of the Child (CRC) for music therapy in paediatric care for children, adolescents, and their families:

Respect for views of the child (Article 12). Children have the right to express their views freely in all matters affecting them, with those views being given due weight according to their age and maturity.

Right to Participation (Article 12)

Freedom of Expression (Article 13). Children have the right to seek, receive, and impart information and ideas of all kinds, including through artistic expression.

Right to Protection from Harm (Article 19)

Health and Health Services (Article 24). Children have the right to the highest attainable standard of health, including mental health services.

(*continued*)

V. Krüger, K. M. Murphy, *Child-Centred Music Therapy*,
https://doi.org/10.1007/978-3-031-85724-9_7

(continued)
Right to Education (Article 28). Children child to education, and with a view to achieving this right progressively and on the basis of equal opportunity (…).

Right to Play and Cultural Activities (Article 31). Children have the right rest and leisure, to engage in play and recreational activities appropriate to the age of the child and to participate freely in cultural life and the arts.

Right to Play, Leisure, and Culture (Article 31). Children have the equal opportunities and the right to participate in cultural, artistic, recreational and leisure activity.

In this chapter we will review literature related to music therapy in for children and adolescents in paediatric care, with a special focus on benefits, music experiences, roles, and functions. We will highlight literature showing how music therapy can be used to advocate for the inclusion of music therapy in medical settings, as part of a holistic approach to children's health and well-being. Music therapy in paediatric settings often incorporates elements of play, creative expression, and cultural participation. It can be seen to fulfil children's rights to engage in cultural and artistic activities, even in medical settings.

In general, paediatric medical care can be defined as a specialized branch of healthcare focused on the physical, emotional, and developmental needs of infants, children, and adolescents (PediStat, 2024). It involves a range of medical services, from routine check-ups and vaccinations to the diagnosis and treatment of illnesses, injuries, and chronic conditions. Paediatric care also includes preventive measures, guidance on nutrition and growth, and support for mental and emotional health, ensuring that children develop healthily and receive appropriate care tailored to their age and specific needs. This care is provided by paediatricians, nurses, and other healthcare professionals such as music therapy trained to address the unique challenges and conditions that affect children.

Music Therapy in Medical Care

Music therapy is considered an integrative treatment designed to facilitate recovery and well-being. Music therapists work in both inpatient and outpatient medical areas, but primarily in high acuity areas such as the paediatric and neonatal intensive care units, and haematology/oncology unit (Knott et al., 2020). Primary goal areas are related to (1) coping with hospitalization, (2) managing pain and anxiety, (3) providing opportunities for emotional expression, (4) sensory stimulation, and (5) normalizing the hospital environment (Ayson, 2008; Tabinowski, 2013). There is a growing body of evidence that supports the inclusion of music therapy in paediatric health care (Stegemann et al., 2019). In this chapter we will highlight those findings that demonstrate congruence between current clinical practice and the UNCRC (1989).

Shoemark et al. (2018) developed a conceptual framework for music therapy in acute paediatric medical care. This framework emerged from a collaborative effort to enhance the understanding and application of music therapy in their acute paediatric context. The team recognized that while articulating the non-musical benefits of music therapy, they often overlooked the patient's unique musical potential, which they identified as a crucial mediator between referral reasons and effective outcomes. The framework articulates three key constructs: the role of music in the patient's life, cultural and contextual influences, and musical manifestations. This framework was subsequently validated through a clinical audit, affirming its inclusivity and effectiveness. Beyond its theoretical contributions, the project exemplifies how interdisciplinary collaboration and reflexive practice can foster a unified approach to service delivery in complex healthcare settings.

Văduva and Balla (2019) investigated the effects of music therapy on emotional optimization of children diagnosed with chronic diseases. Over nine months, 20 children participated in music therapy sessions that involved improvisation, passive listening, rhythmic grounding, and composition. Each session was tailored to individual needs based on age, temperament, diagnosis, and goals, consistent with Article 12 of the UNCRC (1989). Key findings suggest that fear, agitation, and fury were interrelated, while joy emerged as a pivotal variable influencing other aspects like touch, eye brightness, and body language. The results suggest that music therapy positively impacts children with progressive chronic conditions, advocating for its broader implementation and further development.

Benefits of Music Therapy for Children and Adolescents Experiencing Short- or Long-Term Health Issues

Emotional Expression and Coping: Music therapy provides a safe space for children to express their emotions, which can be particularly important for those who may find it difficult to articulate their feelings verbally. Through music, they can process their experiences and develop coping strategies.

Pain Management: Music therapy has been shown to reduce the perception of pain and discomfort in medical settings. Techniques such as guided imagery with music, rhythmic entrainment, and active music-making can help distract from pain and promote relaxation.

Stress Reduction: The hospital environment can be stressful for children and adolescents. Music therapy can create a calming atmosphere, reduce anxiety, and provide a sense of control and predictability.

Social Interaction and Support: Group music therapy sessions can foster social connections and provide peer support. These interactions can help children feel less isolated and more understood by others who share similar experiences.

Enhancing Quality of Life: Engaging in music therapy can bring joy, creativity, and a sense of accomplishment. It can help children maintain a sense of identity and normalcy, contributing to their overall well-being.

General Considerations

Music therapy can provide emotional support, enhance coping strategies, and foster a sense of control for children facing serious medical conditions (Loewy, 2015). Engaging in musical activities allows children to express their emotions and regain a sense of normalcy amidst the challenges of intensive medical treatments Yinger and Lownds (2018). There are many evidence-based protocols that music therapists can refer to for guidance when working with children and adolescents with a reminder that (1) any music experience chosen to meet a treatment goal must be consistent with the values, needs, and preferences of the child or adolescent, and (2) children and adolescents should have a voice as to whether or not to participate in music therapy or the music experiences being offered.

Robb and Carpenter (2009) identified ten music-based interventions reported in the literature that have been used with paediatric patients including breathing entrainment, imagery, music-assisted relaxation, songwriting, lyric analysis, movement, vocal and instrumental re-creation, music listening. These music-based interventions are used in inpatient medical settings (including the paediatric and neonatal intensive care units) and outpatient settings. Yinger and Lownds (2018) then identified how each has been used in paediatric medical care. The use of these interventions will be described in subsequent sectins of this chapter.

Procedural Support

Procedural support is defined as "the use of music and aspects of the therapy relationship to promote healthy coping and decrease distress in individuals undergoing medical procedures" (Ghetti, 2012, p. 6). Beer and Lee (2017) expand upon this definition adding "the music used is designed to specifically address a patient's needs including reducing anxiety and pain perception and to encourage healthy coping behaviors" (p. 266).

Music therapy in paediatric settings involves various activities tailored to meet the developmental, emotional, and medical needs of children. These activities are designed to promote healing, provide comfort, and help children cope with the challenges they face in a hospital or clinical environment. Here are some common music therapy activities used with children in paediatric settings:

1. **Singing and Vocalization**
   - **Sing-alongs**: Encouraging children to sing familiar songs can help in expressing emotions, improving mood, and providing a sense of normalcy.
   - **Songwriting**: Children may create their own songs, which can be therapeutic for expressing feelings or telling their story.
   - **Vocal improvisation**: Spontaneous singing or sound-making to allow for creative expression and communication.
2. **Instrument Play**
   - **Percussion instruments**: Drums, tambourines, and shakers are often used to let children express themselves rhythmically.
   - **Melodic instruments**: Instruments like xylophones, keyboards, or even simple bells may be used to create soothing melodies or for interactive music-making.
   - **Improvisation**: Children may engage in free-form playing, which allows for self-expression and can be a way to explore and process emotions.
3. **Listening to Music**
   - **Live or recorded music**: Therapists might play music that is calming, familiar, or stimulating, depending on the child's needs.
   - **Guided imagery with music**: Combining music with visualization exercises can help in relaxation and pain management.
   - **Music appreciation**: Discussing and analysing the music listened to can help children connect with their emotions and experiences.
4. **Movement to Music**
   - **Dance and movement**: Encouraging children to move to the music can help with physical rehabilitation, coordination, and emotional expression.

(*continued*)

(continued)

- **Parachute play**: Using a parachute in a group setting with music can encourage movement, cooperation, and fun.
- **Musical games**: Activities like musical chairs or freeze dance can be adapted to the child's physical abilities and therapeutic goals.

5. **Music and Art Integration**
   - **Drawing to music**: Children may be asked to draw or paint in response to the music they hear, helping them express emotions visually.
   - **Storytelling with music**: Music can be used to enhance storytelling activities, helping children to connect with the narrative and express themselves.
6. **Interactive Music Making**
   - **Group music sessions**: These foster social interaction, cooperation, and a sense of community among children.
   - **Call-and-response activities**: Encouraging children to respond musically to a prompt can enhance communication and social engagement.
   - **Musical storytelling**: Creating or participating in stories with musical elements can be engaging and therapeutic.
7. **Songwriting**
   - **Lyric analysis**: Discussing the lyrics of songs can help children articulate feelings and process difficult emotions.
   - **Music journaling**: Keeping a journal where they write about how specific music makes them feel or the memories it evokes.
   - **Mood matching**: Selecting or creating music that matches or contrasts with their current emotional state to help with emotional regulation.

Music-based interventions have been used to support paediatric patients undergoing a myriad of medical procedures with one of the earliest published studies by Chetta in 1981. Chetta investigated the effect of music and desensitization on pre-operative anxiety in children. Music therapists and other health care are still researching the effect of music-based interventions on (1) pre-operative anxiety (e.g. Giordano et al., 2020), (2) post-operative pain (e.g. Nilsson et al., 2009), and (3) pain and anxiety related to lumbar puncture (Nhan Nguyen et al., 2010) and vaccinations (e.g. Noguchi, 2006). Music-based interventions have also been used while children are undergoing bone marrow transplants (Burns et al., 2009) and EEG testing (e.g. Loewy et al., 2013)

Two recent systematic reviews summarize the research findings related to the use of music interventions for procedural support. Yinger and Gooding (2015) investigated the efficacy of music-based interventions used to reduce pain and anxiety in adults and children undergoing medical procedures. Eight of the studies included in their review involved procedural support with children and adolescents. A majority of the studies included have a high risk of bias and inadequate intervention reporting. Most of the included studies reported significant reductions in pain and anxiety. Similarly, Kim and Stegemann (2016) investigated the use of music listening for paediatric patients in both clinical and non-clinical settings. The results of their systematic review suggest that music listening in both these settings may reduce pain perception and anxiety; however, the quality of the evidence varied. These results suggest that music-based interventions may reduce pain and anxiety, but more research is needed.

Article 19 of the UNCRC refers to the protection from harm. The research cited above suggests that music-based interventions can minimize both pain and anxiety paediatric patients may experience related to medical procedures they must undergo to maintain their health. Music therapists need to continue to advocate for the inclusion of music therapy when a paediatric patient is undergoing a painful and anxiety-producing procedure.

Music Therapy in Paediatric Oncology

Paediatric oncology is a specialized branch of medicine focused on diagnosing and treating cancer in children. This field addresses the unique needs of young patients, as childhood cancers often differ from those seen in adults in terms of types, behaviour, and response to treatment. Music therapy's role in paediatric oncology has been extensively studied, with numerous findings supporting its positive impact on children's physiological psychological well-being during cancer treatment.

Treatment goals and music therapy methods used in paediatric oncology are like those in other areas of medical music therapy practice.

Common goals addressed include mitigation of pain perception, alleviating anxiety, expression of feelings, improving mood and self-esteem, encourage use of motor and cognitive skills, increase comfort, and provide emotional support (Ghetti & Walker, 2008). In addition, music therapists provide opportunities for mastery and control in an environment where children have little say in what they are experiencing. A comprehensive description of music therapy methods used in paediatric oncology settings may be found in Dun, 2013.

Paediatric oncology patients undergoing haematopoietic stem cell transplants experience extreme stress due to the intensity of the procedure and isolation required (cite). Uggla et al. (2016) investigated the effect of twice-weekly music therapy group participation on heart rate. Increased heart rate is considered a biomarker of stress. Results indicated a significant decrease in evening heart rates that was sustained for 4–8 hours for patients in the music therapy group as compared to the control group. In a follow-up study involving 29 patients aged 0–17 years, Uggla et al. (2018) reported an improvement in the children's self-reported health-related quality of life (HRQoL) following individual music therapy. Notably, physical functioning in the music therapy group improved significantly by the time of discharge (adjusted $p = 0.04$). Additionally, patients receiving music therapy reported less signs of treatment anxiety and worry at the time of discharge. Patients in the control group received music therapy once they were discharged from the hospital. Patients in the control group showed improved results in all domains measured by the HRQoL.

Knoerl et al. (2023) investigated the experiences of adolescent and young adult cancer patients who participated in a mindfulness-based music therapy intervention before and during the COVID-19 pandemic. Sixteen participants, aged 20–39, were interviewed about their experiences with both in-person and virtual delivery of the therapy. The results revealed that while virtual sessions were feasible, participants faced challenges like finding private spaces and generally preferred the in-person format, which fostered a stronger sense of connection with the music and family members. Both formats, however, were effective in promoting relaxation and reducing anxiety and stress. The study highlights the importance of considering contextual factors in future music therapy designs.

Helander et al. (2020) interviewed caregivers, hospital volunteers, and members of the medical team working on an ambulatory chemotherapy unit to explore their experiences and descriptions of the impact of music therapy interventions on the children, the hospital environment, the caregivers, and the interviewees themselves. Twelve themes emerged from the interviews, with attention, enjoyment, and relaxation being the key themes to describe the benefits of music therapy from their perception. They reported that between and during medical procedures, active and receptive music therapy interventions provided a supportive distraction from the challenging environment, thereby helping the children to better cope with the situation and providing possibilities to encourage social engagement and interactions. From their perception, the music therapy interventions not only had a positive impact on the children, but also on the people around them and on the atmosphere of the hospital environment. Through music therapy, children's cooperation during medical procedures improved, which facilitated the staff in carrying out the procedures. These findings support music therapy as having an ability to create meaningful moments in an intense and high-tempo medical unit and contribute to the child's treatment process from a holistic perspective. However, missing from this study is the perceptions of the children. It is unknown if the children who received treatment in this chemotherapy unit would describe their experiences in the same way as the interviewees. This study is an example of where the voice of the adults providing treatment was dominant and the child's voice was not heard.

Music Therapy in Paediatric Intensive Care Units

The Paediatric Intensive Care Unit (PICU) is a specialized division within hospitals dedicated to the critical care of children with severe or life-threatening medical conditions. These units are staffed by a multidisciplinary team that includes paediatric intensivists[1] (including surgeons and other specialists), nurses, respiratory therapists, and other specialists who possess expertise in paediatric care. The PICU environment is equipped with advanced medical technology designed for use with children from birth through age 18. The PICU serves a critical role in both stabilizing and managing complex medical conditions among children, combining specialized care with the sensitivity required for treating younger patients.

The use of music therapy in paediatric intensive care settings has gained attention, particularly for its physiological and psychological benefits.

[1] Paediatric intensivists are physicians who have completed subspeciality fellowship training in intensive care for children.

Children who require hospitalization in the PICU are at risk for developing maladaptive stress responses possibly related to medical environment, isolation, separation from family, and inability to communicate or even move around (Mata Ferro et al., 2023). Ghetti and Hannan (2008) identify common goal areas as alleviation of anxiety, promoting relaxation, decreasing agitation, improving pain management, increasing sensory stimulation, improving active cognition, alleviating depression, and increasing range of motion (pp. 83–86). A comprehensive description of music therapy methods commonly used in the PICU may be found in Ghetti (2013). Bringing music into this highly technical and often noisy environment can also bring a calming aesthetic that has benefits for patients, families, and staff (Del Olmo et al., 2010; Ghetti, 2013).

The research examining the efficacy of music-based interventions on pain, anxiety, stress responses, or other clinical outcomes for paediatric PICU patients is limited. Del Olmo et al. (2010) investigated the effect of live, improvised vocal music accompanied with keyboard or guitar on infants hospitalized in the PICU. Results indicated significant positive changes in respiration rate and heart rate as compared to the no music condition. In a follow-up study (Del Ormo et al., 2015) the same protocol was used to determine its effect on levels of discomfort. Results indicated a significant positive change in the infant's distress levels. Buzzi et al. (2022) investigated the effect of pre-recorded music on paediatric PICU patient sedation levels as measured by the COMFORT Behavior Scale (CBC). Patients enrolled in the study listened to music that was composed, played, and recorded by two musicians and music therapists for one hour twice a day, once in the morning and again in the afternoon. Results showed a positive reduction in CBC scores after 30 minutes and again at 60 minutes. Mata Ferro et al. (2023) examined the efficacy of live music on the vital signs, pain, and discomfort of paediatric patients in the PICU for management of chronic respiratory illness. Patients enrolled in the study received 10 minutes of live music once a week. The music therapist chose children's songs (both vocal and instrumental) consistent with each patient's age group, interests, and emotional state and in their native language. Results indicated significant positive changes in heart rate, respiration rate, and discomfort. Notable in this study is that the music chosen was in the patient's native language, consistent with Article 8 of the UNCRC (1989) which is related to the right of children to maintain their identity and culture. Taken together these studies suggest that live music, and speciality composted pre-recorded music can have a positive effect on sedation, distress, and vital signs. Clearly more research is needed.

Music Therapy in the Neonatal Intensive Care Unit

The neonatal intensive care unit (NICU) is similar in function to the PICU with the exception that only newborn infants are admitted to the NICU. Infants who need critical care after birth are admitted to the PICU or in some cases the Paediatric Intensive Cardiac Care Unit (PICCU). Newborns are admitted to the NICU primarily because of complications related to premature birth (CDC, 2024). Other reasons for a NICU admission may be related to congenital diagnoses such as heart defects, incomplete closure of the neural tube, gastrointestinal disorders, chromosomal disorders (Smith et al., 2018), complications during pregnancy or delivery (March of Dimes, 2016), and neonatal abstinence syndrome (Siu & Robinson, 2014).

There is a robust body of research that supports the inclusion of music therapy as a treatment modality in the neonatal intensive care unit (NICU). The NICU is a highly technical medical unit that provides care for newborn children who need specialized care due to prematurity or serious medical complications. There are several ways in which music is used in the NICU including multi-modal stimulation with music (Stanley & Walworth, 2010), pacifier-activated lullaby (Stanley & Walworth, 2010), contingent singing (Shoemark, 2013) of kin (Loewy et al., 2013), recreation of womb sounds (Loewy et al., 2013), creative music therapy (Haslbeck, 2013), and recorded sedative music (Calabro & Grocke, 2017). Music therapists may use any or all the methods to meet the immediate medical and developmental needs of the infant. Lullaby singing is used alone or in conjunction with the music therapy methods listed above to minimize pain during procedures (e.g. Ullsten et al., 2017), facilitate sleep (Loewy et al., 2013), improve physiological measures related to stress (Özgürbüz et al., 2024), and improve comfort during feeding (Bağli et al., 2024). A culturally appropriate form of lullaby, *Song of Kin* (developed by Loewy), "is a melody that is identified by a parent that has been used in a family's history or at present that is familiar and/or representative of the culture of that family's community" (Loewy et al., 2013, p. 906).

Environmental Music Therapy in the NICU

Environment music therapy (EMT) is defined as a "human-centered trauma-informed intervention that encompasses utilisation of the metaphoric and associative properties of live music to modulate patients', caregivers, and staff's perception of the hospital milieu as a potentially hostile environment" (Rossetti, 2020, p. 131). When used in the NICU, EMT aims to transform this very technical and noisy unit into a more comforting and healing space.

Noise levels in the NICU often exceed the maximum 45 dB levels recommended by the American Academy of Pediatrics which risk the neurodevelopment of infants. Arnon et al. (2022) investigated and compared the effect of individual music therapy (IMT) and EMT on noise levels in an open bay NICU room. Results indicated that both methods reduced noise in an open bay NICU room. Further, results indicated that the signal-to-noise ratio was higher in the rooms that received music therapy, thus suggesting that these methods may support the neurodevelopment of infants. These findings, though preliminary, are important as Article 19 of the UNCRC should remind health care providers of their obligation to protect children from harm. Both IMT and EMT are prime ways to protect neonates from noise-induced harm.

Family-Centred Care and Music Therapy

Family-centred care is an approach to the delivery of health care that involves partnerships with healthcare providers, patients, and their families. It emphasizes "working with patients and families, rather than just doing 'to' or 'for' them (Institute for Patient- and Family-Centered Care, n.d.). This approach to paediatric medical care is supported by the UNCRC Article 18 which outlines parental responsibilities in supporting their children. There are several examples of parental involvement in music therapy sessions involving paediatric medical settings.

Uggla et al. (2019) explored children and their parents' experiences of the interactive music therapy process during and after hematopoietic stem cell transplantation. Six families (including parents and their children) and the music therapist were interviewed by an independent psychologist. Three themes emerged from this analysis: experiences of competence and self-recognition; interactive affect regulation as a potential for change; and the importance of the therapeutic relationship. This suggests that music therapy was important in both coping and managing the treatment.

Ayson (2008) explored the role of short-term music therapy in supporting children and their parents facing the difficulties of hospitalization by reviewing clinical notes and her reflective journals and conducting semi-structured interviews with the children's parents and staff. The data analysis indicated that music therapy normalized the hospital environment and provided emotional and psychological support for children and elicited positive changes in mood and anxiety. Music therapy also appeared to support the parent-child relationship. Missing from this study is the voice of the child participants through either verbal or non-verbal means of expression. UNCRC Article 14 notes the importance of the child's voice in decisions concerning their well-being. A stronger case of the inclusion of music therapy could have been made, if the author had interviewed the children as well.

Several studies have suggested the positive effects music therapy can have on parent–infant bonding, though not all reported significant results. Ghetti et al. (2023) investigated the impact of parent-led, infant-directed singing, facilitated by a music therapist, on parent–infant bonding in preterm infants. Conducted across five countries in level III and IV NICUs, this randomized clinical trial included 206 preterm infants and their parents, with follow-ups extending to 12 months. The intervention involved singing sessions either during NICU hospitalization or post-discharge, compared to standard care alone. Results showed no significant differences in mother–infant bonding scores at 6 and 12 months between the music therapy and control groups, indicating that while the intervention was safe and well-received, it did not produce clinically significant improvements in bonding. The study highlights the importance of evaluating the effectiveness of such interventions while ensuring their safety and acceptance in clinical settings.

Gaden et al. (2022) evaluated the short-term effects of music therapy for premature infants and their caregivers on mother–infant bonding, and maternal anxiety and depression. Parent–infant dyads in the experimental group received three music therapy sessions per work that involved parent-led singing supported by the music therapist. Significant changes in bonding, maternal depression, or anxiety were not achieved; however, there was high retention of parents in the experimental group, suggesting that research with salutogenic outcomes is warranted.

Epstein et al. (2023) chose a qualitative method to explore the lived experiences of parent who engaged in longer-term music therapy with their pre-term infants spanning in time from birth to six months. Data analysis revealed two important themes: (1) music therapy as a haven and (2) music therapy as enabling integration of music into the parent–infant relationship. The results of this study support Gaden et al.'s (2022) that salutogenic outcomes are warranted to further understand the benefits of parent–infant music therapy.

Gaps in the Research

This limited review of current research into the efficacy of music therapy for children and adolescents with acute, chronic, or life-limiting illness suggests music-based interventions have positive effects on outcomes related to stress, anxiety, mood, and emotional expression. Current research predominantly focuses on a medical model, emphasizing empirical evidence, randomized controlled trials (RCTs), and meta-analyses to justify the effectiveness of music therapy. While valuable, this approach overlooks how music therapy fits within a more holistic, child- and family-centred framework that emphasizes individual experience and personal context. There is a lack of qualitative or mixed method research designs that would provide a deeper, more nuanced understanding of how children, adolescents, and families perceive music therapy's role in their health care.

One significant gap in the research is the limited focus on paediatric populations, as highlighted by Yinger and Gooding's systematic review, which found that only 8 out of 50 studies focused on children and adolescents. More research is needed to explore the specific benefits of music therapy for younger patients undergoing various medical procedures. Additionally, the high risk of bias and inadequate intervention reporting in many studies suggest a need for more rigorous and well-designed research to provide reliable evidence on the effectiveness of music therapy in these settings.

Music therapists often work as part of an interdisciplinary team, yet there is limited research on how medical professionals perceive the benefits of music therapy, or how and why they may make a referral to music therapy for one of their patients. Ways in which members of the interdisciplinary team can collaborate to improve outcomes should also be explored.

While music therapy is recognized for fostering emotional expression, there is a gap in understanding how it can specifically contribute to building coping mechanisms and resilience in children and adolescents with chronic and life-limiting illnesses. Finally, there is a need for more research on the ethical considerations of involving children and adolescents in music therapy, especially regarding consent, autonomy, and the role of family in therapy settings. Addressing these gaps can provide a more comprehensive understanding of music therapy's role in paediatric medical care and help tailor interventions to meet the diverse needs of this population.

The integration of family-centred care in music therapy, particularly for premature infants, highlights the importance of involving parents in therapeutic processes. However, more research is needed to understand the long-term effects of such interventions and their impact on both infants and caregivers. Additionally, the application of music therapy in broader medical settings, including substance use disorders and other chronic conditions, remains underexplored and could benefit from more interdisciplinary studies.

Overall, addressing these research gaps can provide a more comprehensive understanding of the role of music therapy in surgical and procedural settings, leading to more effective and evidence-based interventions that can enhance patient outcomes and well-being.

Recommendations for Research

While the existing literature provides strong evidence for the efficacy of music therapy in paediatric medical settings, some methodological limitations must be addressed in future research. Many studies rely on small sample sizes, limiting the generalizability of their findings. Additionally, incomplete documentation of each music-based intervention used (such as the type of music used, the duration of sessions, qualifications of the interventionist) makes it difficult to standardize treatment protocols.

It is essential for medical music therapy research to adopt an integrative medicine framework that moves away from the traditional medical model to meet the spirit of the UNCRC and to meet research gaps in music therapy for paediatric medical care. This involves integrating a child- and family-centred approach into research designs that emphasizes individual experiences and personal contexts. In this way, music therapists will be able to use research findings to assist with a "best interest of the child determination" in their clinical work to. The following recommendations for research are offered as a starting point:

1. More research should be done with children, rather than on children.
2. Future studies should focus on larger-scale RCTs with standardized protocols to strengthen the evidence base and explore the integration of music therapy into routine paediatric healthcare.
3. Longitudinal studies are needed to explore long-term impact of music therapy as well as to learn if, and how therapeutic benefits evolve over time.
4. Researchers should be explicit when describing music-based interventions following the guidelines developed by Robb et al.
5. Researchers should continue to build upon the research that has been done while also broadening the scope of diagnoses and psychosocial outcomes.
6. Family-cantered music therapy should continue, again broadening the scope of settings, diagnoses, and age range of patients.
7. Mechanistic clinical trials are needed to understand the mechanism of action for music-based interventions.

References

Arnon, S., Epstein, S., Ghetti, C., Bauer-Rusek, S., Taitelbaum-Swead, R., & Yakobson, D. (2022). Music therapy intervention in an open bay neonatal intensive care unit room is associated with less noise and higher signal to noise ratios: A case-control study. *Children, 9*, 1187. https://doi.org/10.3390/children9081187

Ayson, C. (2008). Child-parent wellbeing in a paediatric ward: The role of music therapy in supporting children and their parents facing the challenge of hospitalisation. *Voices: A World Forum for Music Therapy, 8*(1). https://doi.org/10.15845/voices.v8i1.449

Bağli, E., Küçükoğlu, S., & Soylu, H. (2024). The effect of lullabies and classical music on preterm neonates' cerebral oxygenation, vital signs, and comfort during orogastric tube feeding: A randomized controlled trial. *Biological Research for Nursing, 26*(2), 181–191. https://doi.org/10.1177/10998004231202404

Beer, L. E., & Lee, K. (2017). Music therapy and procedural support: Defining and identifying areas of practice. *Music and Medicine, 9*(4), 262–267.

Burns, D. S., Robb, S. L., & Haase, J. E. (2009). Exploring the feasibility of a therapeutic music video intervention in adolescents and young adults during stem-cell transplantation. *Cancer Nursing, 32*(5), E8–E16. https://doi.org/10.1097/NCC.0b013e3181a4802c

Buzzi, F., Yahya, N. B., Gambazza, S., Binda, F., Galazzi, A., Ferrari, A., Crespan, S., Al-Atroushy, H. A., Cantoni, B. M., Laquintana, D., & Collaborative Group. (2022). Use of musical intervention in the pediatric intensive care unit of a developing country: A pilot pre–post study. *Children, 9*, 455. https://doi.org/10.3390/children9040455

Calabro, J., & Grocke, D. E. (2017). Music therapy for infants with neonatal abstinence syndrome. *Music & Medicine, 9*(1), 37–44.

Center for Disease Control and Prevention (CDC). (2024, October 8). *About adverse childhood experiences*. https://www.cdc.gov/aces/about/

Del Olmo, M. J., Rodríguez, C., & Ruza, F. (2010). Music therapy in the PICU: 0- to 6-month-old babies. *Music and Medicine, 2*(3), 158–166.

Del Ormo, M. J., Tarrio, F. R., Garrido, C. R., & marina, P. C. (2015). The effects of a music therapy intervention in PICU as measured by the comfort behavior scale. *Music and Medicine, 7*(2), 20–24.

Dun, B. (2013). Children with cancer. In J. Bradt (Ed.), *Guidelines for music therapy practice in pediatric care* (pp. 292–323). Barcelona Publishers.

Epstein, S., Elefant, C., Arnon, S., & Ghetti, C. (2023). Music therapy spanning from NICU to home: An interpretative phenomenological analysis of Israeli parents' experiences in the LongSTEP trial. *Nordic Journal of Music Therapy, 32*(5), 373–396. https://doi.org/10.1080/08098131.2023.2180773

Gaden, T. S., Ghetti, C., Kvestad, I., Bieleninik, Ł., Størksen Stordal, A., Assmus, J., Arnon, S., Elefant, C., Ettenberger, M., Lichtensztejn, M., Manger-snes, J., Janner Røed, C., Vederhus, B. J., & Gold, C. (2022). Short-term music therapy for families with premature infants: A randomized trial. *Pediatrics, 149*(2), e2021052797.

Ghetti, C. M. (2012). Music therapy as procedural support for invasive medical procedures: Towards the development of music therapy theory. *Nordic Journal of Music Therapy, 2*(11), 3–35. https://doi.org/10.1080/08098131.2011.571278

Ghetti, C. M. (2013). Pediatric intensive care. In J. Bradt (Ed.), *Guidelines for music therapy practice in pediatric care* (pp. 152–204). Barcelona Publishers.

Ghetti, C., & Hannan, A. (2008). Pediatric intensive care unit. In D. Hanson-Abromeit & C. Colwell (Eds.), *Music therapy for pediatrics in hospital settings* (pp. 71–106). American Music Therapy Association.

Ghetti, C., & Walker, J. (2008). Hematology, oncology, and bone-marrow transplant. In D. Hanson-Abromeit & C. Colwell (Eds.), *Music therapy for pediatrics in hospital settings* (pp. 147–193). American Music Therapy Association.

Ghetti, C. M., Gaden, T. S., Bieleninik, L., Kvestad, I., Assmus, J., Stordal, A. S., Aristizabal Sanchez, L. F., Arnon, S., Dulsrud, J., Elefant, C., Epstein, S., Ettenberger, M., Glosli, H., Konieczna-Nowak, L., Lichtensztejn, M., Lindvall, M. W., Mangersnes, J., Murcia Fernández, L. D., Røed, C. J., Saá, G., van Roy, B., Vederhus, B. J., & Gold, C. (2023). Effect of music therapy on parent-infant bonding among infants born preterm: A randomized clinical trial. *JAMA Network Open, 6*(5), e2315750. https://doi.org/10.1001/jamanetworkopen.2023.15750

Giordano, F., Zanchi, B., De Leonardis, F., Rutigliano, C., Esposito, F., Brienza, N., & Santoro, N. (2020). The influence of music therapy on preoperative anxiety in pediatric oncology patients undergoing invasive procedures. *The Arts in Psychotherapy,* 68. https://s443-doi-org.libdatabase.newpaltz.edu/10.1016/j.aip.2020.101649

Haslbeck, F. B. (2013). Creative music therapy with premature infants: An analysis of video footage. *Nordic Journal of Music Therapy, 23*(1), 5–31. https://doi.org/10.1080/08098131.2013.780091

Helander, S., Gattino, G. S., & Baumann, E. (2020). How music therapy is perceived in a pediatric outpatient chemotherapy unit in a Peruvian hospital: Report of an experience. *Revista Brasileira de Musicoterapia, 22*(29), 36–52. https://doi.org/10.51914/brjmt.29.2020.387

Kim, J., & Stegemann, T. (2016). Music listening for children and adolescents in health care contexts: A systematic review. *The Arts in Psychotherapy, 51,* 72–85. https://s443-doiorg.libdatabase.newpaltz.edu/10.1016/j.aip.2016.08.007

Knoerl, R., Mazzola, E., Woods, H., Buchbinder, E., Frazier, L., laCasce, A., Luskin, M. R., Phillips, C. S., Thornton, K., Berry, D. L., & Ligibel, J. (2023). Exploring influencing factors of anxiety improvement following mindfulness=based music therapy in young adults with cancer. *Journal of Music Therapy, 60*(2), 131–148. https://doi.org/10.1093/jmt/thac017

Knott, D., Biard, M., Nelson, K. E., Epstein, S., Robb, S. L., & Ghetti, C. M. (2020). A survey of music therapists working in pediatric medical settings in the United States. *Journal of Music Therapy, 57*(1), 34–65. https://doi.org/10.1093/jmt/thz019

Loewy, J. (2015). Medical music therapy for children. In B. L. Wheeler (Ed.), *Music therapy handbook* (pp. 425–440). The Guilford Press.

Loewy, J., Steward, K., Dassler, A.-M., Telsy, A., & Homel, P. (2013). The effects of music therapy on vital signs, feeding, and sleep in premature infants. *Pediatrics, 131*(5), 902–908. https://doi.org/10.1542/peds.2012-1367

March of Dimes. (2016). *Peristats.* Retrieved from http://www.marchofdimes.org/peristats/whatsnew.aspx?id=42

Mata Ferro, M., Falcó-Pegueroles, A., Fernández-Lorenzo, R., Saz-Roy, M. A., Rodríguez-Forner, O., Estrada Jurado, C. M., Bonet Julià, N., Geli Benito, C., Hernádez Hernáde, R., & Bosch Alcaraz, A. (2023). The effect of a live music therapy intervention on critically ill paediatric patients in the intensive care unit: A quasi-experimental pretest-posttest study. *Australian Critical Care, 36*(6), 967–973. https://doi.org/10.1016/j.aucc.2023.01.006

Nhan Nguyen, T., Nilsson, S., Hellström, A.-L., & Bengtson, A. (2010). Music therapy to reduce pain and anxiety in children with cancer undergoing lumbar puncture: A randomized clinical trial. *Journal of Pediatric Oncology Nursing, 27*(3), 146–155.

Nilsson, S., Kokinsky, E., Nilsson, U., Sidenvall, B., & Enskär, K. (2009). School-aged children's experience of postoperative music medicine on pain, distress and anxiety. *Pediatric Anesthesia, 19*, 1184–1190.

Noguchi, L. K. (2006). The effect of music versus nonmusic on behavioral signs of distress and self-report of pain in pediatric injection patients. *Journal of Music Therapy, 43*, 16–38.

Özgürbüz, N., Bahar, A., Tuna, A., & Çopur, E. (2024). The effect of lullaby played to preterm infants in neonatal intensive care units on physiological parameters and pain. *Journal of Pediatric Nursing, 79*, 133–140. https://doi.org/10.1016/j.pedn.2024.08.019

PediStat. (2024, July 1). *What is the age range for pediatrics?* https://www.pedistat.com/blog/what-the-age-range-for-pediatrics

Robb, S. L., & Carpenter, J. S. (2009). A review of music-based intervention reporting in pediatrics. *Journal of Health Psychology, 14*(4), 490–501. https://doi.org/10.1177/1359105309103568

Rossetti, A. (2020). Environmental Music Therapy (EMT): Music's contribution to changing hospital atmospheres and perceptions of environments. *Music and Medicine, 12*(2), 130–141. https://s443-doiorg.libdatabase.newpaltz.edu/10.47513/mmd.v12i2.742

Shoemark, H. (2013). Full term hospitalized newborns. In J. Bradt (Ed.), *Guidelines for music therapy practice in pediatric care* (pp. 116–151). Barcelona Publishers.

Shoemark, H., Rimmer, J., Bower, J., Tucquet, B., Miller, L., Fisher, M., Ogburn, N., & Dun, B. (2018). A conceptual framework: The musical self as a unique pathway to outcomes in the acute pediatric health setting. *Journal of Music Therapy, 55*(1), 1–26. https://doi.org/10.1093/jmt/thx018

Siu, A., & Robinson, C. A. (2014). Neonatal abstinence syndrome: essentials for the practitioner. *The Journal of Pediatric Pharmacology and Therapeutics : JPPT: The Official Journal of PPAG, 19*(3), 147–155. https://s443-doiorg.libdatabase.newpaltz.edu/10.5863/1551-6776-19.3.147

Smith, A., Caine, K., & Hanson-Abromeit, D. (2018). Music therapy for neonatal intensive care. In A. Knight, B. laGasse, & A. Clair (Eds.), *Music therapy: An Introduction to the profession* (pp. 247–264). American Music Therapy Association.

Stanley, J. M., & Walworth, D. (2010). *Music therapy with premature infants: Research and developmental interventions* (2nd ed.). American Music Therapy Association.

Stegemann, T., Geretsegger, M., Phan Quoc, E., Riedl, H., & Smetana, M. (2019). Music therapy and other music-based interventions in pediatric health care: An overview. *Medicine, 6*(1), 25. https://doi.org/10.3390/medicines6010025

Tabinowski, K. (2013). *A survey of current music therapy practices in pediatric hospitals and units* [Unpublished master's thesis]. Florida State University.

Uggla, L., Bonde, L. O., Svahn, B. M., et al. (2016). Music therapy can lower the heart rates of severely sick children. *Acta Paediatrica, 105*(11), 1225–1230. https://doi.org/10.1111/apa.13452

Uggla, L., Bonde, L.-O., Hammar, U., Wrangsjo, B., & Gustafsson, B. (2018). Music therapy supported the health-related quality of life for children undergoing haematopoietic stem cell transplants. *Acta Paediatrica, 107*, 1986–1994. https://doi.org/10.1111/apa.14515

Uggla, L., Mårtenson Blom, K., Bonde, L. O., et al. (2019). An explorative study of qualities in interactive processes with children and their parents in music therapy during and after pediatric hematopoietic stem cell transplantation. *Medicine, 6*(1), 28. https://doi.org/10.3390/medicines6010028

Ullsten, A., Eriksson, M., Klässbo, M., & Volgsten, U. (2017). Live music therapy with lullaby singing as affective support during painful procedures: A case study with microanalysis. *Nordic Journal of Music Therapy, 26*(2), 142–166. http://dx.doi.org/10.1080/08098131.2015.1131187

United Nations. (1989). *Convention on the rights of the child*. https://www.ohchr.org/en/instruments-mechanisms/instruments/convention-rights-child

Văduva, L. P., & Balla, A. (2019). A study of the efficiency of music therapy, art and play therapy on hospitalized children diagnosed with chronic illnesses. *Studia Universitatis Babes-Bolvai-Musica, 64*(2), 147–160.

Yinger, O. S., & Gooding, L. F. (2015). A systematic review of music-based intervention for procedural support. *Journal of Music Therapy, 52*(1), 1–77. https://doi.org/10.1093/jmt/thv004

Yinger, O. S., & Lownds, K. (2018). Music therapy in pediatric medicine. In A. Knight, B. LaGasse, & A. Clair (Eds.), *Music therapy: An Introduction to the profession* (pp. 265–280). American Music Therapy Association.

PART III

Advancing Ethical and Child-Centered Research

CHAPTER 8

Music Therapy Research and the Best Interest of the Child

> **"A primary consideration"**
>
> "The best interest of the child" principle shall be "a primary consideration" which provides for special protection of children in any context and acknowledges their unique vulnerability. The principle is of non-derogable nature, which means it does not allow for limitations even in times of emergencies (UN Committee on the Rights of the Child, 2013).

Introduction

Evidence-based practice is considered the gold standard for determining whether music therapy services should be part of the education and health care of individuals across the life span. Evidence-based practice in its truest form can be considered an iterative process in which the music therapist considers the best available research,[1] their practice wisdom and individuals' preferences when making decisions about the use of music experiences to meet treatment goals. The published research in peer-reviewed music therapy journals is not as robust when it comes to studies in which children are the participants. This omission in the literature creates an ethical

[1] Research is defined to mean all forms of scientific inquiry including quantitative, qualitative, and descriptive research methods.

V. Krüger, K. M. Murphy, *Child-Centred Music Therapy*,
https://doi.org/10.1007/978-3-031-85724-9_8

challenge that may prevent music therapists from making treatment decisions that are in the best interest of the child. The purpose of this chapter then is to review the ethical issues related to conducting research remembering that the best "rights of the child" shall be a primary consideration in all actions related to research in which children are participants.

Research Ethics: Brief Overview

From Article 19:

Assessment of the child's best interests must also include consideration of the child's safety, that is, the right of the child to protection against all forms of physical or mental violence, injury, or abuse (Article 19). For researchers this means that all research involving children will meet or exceed all ethical requirements or guidelines.

Historically, children, especially those with disabilities, were often participants in medical research without their assent or parental consent. For example, the radiation studies conducted in the 1940s in which institutionalized children were given radioactive iron (West, 1998). Similarly, in the 1960s children living in a state institution were intentionally infected with the hepatitis virus without their assent. Additionally, parents were not given accurate information about the study prior to giving consent. These two examples, while extreme, highlight the need for protection of children who participate in research.

There are several documents that outline the essentials of ethical research practices when children are participants. These include the Belmont Report (National Commission for the Protection of Human Subjects, 1979), General Data Protection Regulation (Regulation (EU) 2016/679, 2016), The World Medical Association (2013), and the World Health Organization (n.d.). Common ethical principles among these documents are respect for persons, beneficence, and justice. Each of these principles will be defined and discussed as they pertain to research with children.

Respect for Persons

The principle of respect for persons is grounded in the concepts of autonomy and self-determination. According to *Merriam-Webster* (n.d.), the "kids" definition of autonomy is "the power or right of self-government." In medical settings autonomy is considered "the quality or state of being independent, free, and self-directing" (Merriam-Webster, n.d.). We see elements of both these definitions when we consider the meaning of autonomy as it relates to respect for persons.

Respect for persons has two components: (1) individuals who are invited to participate in research have autonomy, and (2) those with diminished capacity to make autonomous decisions are afforded extra protection (e.g. National Commission for the Protection of Human Subjects of Biomedical and Behavioral Research, 1979). In research, autonomy guarantees the right participants have for self-governance as it were. This means participants are given the ability to freely decide whether to participate in a research study after having time to carefully consider the risks and benefits and without coercion. Additionally, they have the right to withdraw at any time without penalty or prejudice.

The second component of the definition requires that extra protection be put in place for individuals who may not have capacity for self-governing. The ability to self-govern matures over an individual's life and may at some point diminish due to "illness, mental disability, or circumstances that severely restrict liberty" (National Commission for the Protection of Human Subjects of Biomedical and Behavioral Research, 1979, p. 5). The potential for harm and level of benefit should determine the level of protection afforded potential research participants. The capacity for autonomy, or self-governance, should periodically be re-evaluated as the status of a person with diminished capacity may change over time (National Commission for the Protection of Human Subjects of Biomedical and Behavioral Research, 1979).

Beneficence

Beneficence is generally understood to mean doing good beyond what is expected. The Hippocratic Oath, estimated to be written around 400 BC, reminds researchers to *first do no harm* (Miles, 2004). It is this concept of not doing harm that underlies the first principle of beneficence. One only must review the storied history of research to recall that many research participants endured pain, mental anguish, disease, and even death to understand the importance of beneficence. Further, researchers are required to maximize the benefits of their research while reducing harm. This is done through a careful and thorough evaluation of the risks and benefits of a research protocol. The potential benefits of a research study must outweigh the risks.

The notion that music therapy research has more than minimal risk needs to be carefully considered in intervention studies. As an example, songwriting is a common music experience used to facilitate emotional expression. This method has the potential to amplify emotions and re-traumatize a child or adolescent. In this case, the principle of beneficence reminds researchers that a thorough history of each participant's background is necessary to prevent re-traumatization. Other factors that should be taken into consideration are the child's developmental level, strengths, and challenges as they relate to the music intervention being studied.

Justice

The third principle to consider is that of justice which was first identified in the Belmont Report (Pieper & Thomson, 2013). The Commissioners cited several examples of injustice in their report noting that historically the burden of research fell to poor hospitalized patients with the benefits being provided to the wealthy. Other examples included the forced inclusion of prisoners in Nazi concentration camps and the Tuskegee syphilis study. Since the publication of the Belmont report, other countries have included a discussion about justice in research (Pieper & Thomson, 2013; Pratt et al. 2020).

The principle of justice refers to the fair and equitable distribution of the benefits, as well as the risks related to research. There is not a general definition of fairness as it relates to the distribution of risks and benefits related to research (Mastroiann et al. 1994), but the Belmont Report (National Commission for the Protection of Human Subjects of Biomedical and Behavioral Research, 1979) offers the following guidance: (1) research participants should be selected as they are "directly related to the problem being studied" (p. 6) and (2) members of their group will have access to and benefit from the research study's results.

The second issue highlights a significant limitation in music therapy: the lack of access to services for many of the populations from which research participants are drawn. This is a global challenge, as music therapy remains inaccessible to most people worldwide. The dilemma lies in the fact that, without a robust evidence base, music therapy is often perceived as optional rather than a necessary therapeutic service. To address this, music therapists must take a more active role in advocating for broader access to music therapy services in order to promote justice and equity in both research opportunities and access to promising music therapy treatments.

Research Ethics: Applications to Research with Children

Article 5 of the UNCRC

- The nature of the relationship between children and their parents should evolve as the child matures.

Article 12 of the UNCRC

- Ensures that children capable of forming and expressing their views should be afforded the right to do so.
- Their views should be acknowledged in the context of their age and maturity.

Article 13 of the UNCRC

- Ensures that children have the right to express themselves using appropriate methods.

Ethical research guidelines from most countries, the WHO, GDPR, and the Belmont report do not prohibit children from participating in research. They do, however, consider children in need of extra protection as they are presumed incapable of self-determination (Belmont Report; Part B, Sec B, para. 4) or do not have decisional capacity.[2] Children are asked to give assent to participate in research, when possible, but in most countries, parents or legal guardians must give consent for their child to participate.

[2] Decisional capacity involves "understanding, appreciation, reasoning, and the ability to express a choice" (Grisso & Applebaum, 1998; Roth et al., 1977).

The issue of informed consent versus assent for children and adolescents is being debated among research ethicists, medical professionals, and researchers (e.g. Hein et al., 2015). Some scholars view children as having the experience and capacity to make informed decisions as to whether to participate in research (Chakraborty et al., 2012). This sentiment is supported by Crane and Broome (2017) findings that most children have “the ability to understand essential elements of research, although there is variability in children’s level of understanding” (p. 200). It has been recommended that a child/adolescent’s decisional capacity be evaluated when determining if they are competent to make an informed decision with regard to participation in a research study. Further, this assessment should be used to determine if a child’s assent or refusal to participate in a research study should be given more weight than parental consent or refusal. Chenneville (2023) suggests that assessing a child’s decisional capacity may lead to “improved adherence to research protocols” which will result in more reliable research results.

There are valid tools to measure the decisional capacity of children with the MacArthur Competence Assessment Tool for Treatment being used most frequently (Applebaum, 2007). This assessment tool includes a structured interview that includes information related to the specific decision to be made.

Supporting the rights of children who are determined to have decisional capacity is often thwarted by protectionist ethical frameworks in which they are considered vulnerable, and at risk, or by developing child models that consider minors to be incapable of making an informed decision (Chakraborty et al., 2012), These models remove agency and autonomy from a child giving sole authority for participation in a research study to the parent/guardian. Articles 12 and 13 of the UNCRC remind researchers that children who have decisional capacity have the right to be heard and should be allowed to make decisions about their involvement in research (Krappmann, 2010). These authors challenge researchers to see children as “active agents endowed with capacities to contribute” (Chakraborty et al., 2012). Further, they are encouraged to actively listen to and give weight to the concerns children may have regarding research participation (Krappman, 2010).

Ethical Research with Children

Article 24 of the UNCRC

- Children are entitled to enjoy the highest standards of health.

Excluding children from music therapy research may prevent them from enjoying the "highest standards of health" as required by the UNCRC and subject them to music therapy methods and protocols that have been developed for adults. Involving children in research comes with additional oversight as they are often considered vulnerable, incapable of making informed decisions, and in need of extra oversight and protection. As noted by Powell and Smith (2009), children are beginning to be seen as active participants in research given developments in childhood studies (p. 124). There is a growing call to involving children in research (e.g. Sinclair, 2004). Music therapy researchers should heed this call as participation will better inform music therapy treatment for children while upholding the principle of justice.

Music therapists are encouraged to evaluate the decisional capacity of children rather than excluding their voices entirely in deciding whether they wish to participate. Chenneville (2023) describes two ethical models that music therapy researchers can consider when inviting children to participate in a research study: the Goodness-of-Fit Ethical Framework proposed by Fisher (2003) and the Protection-Autonomy Model proposed by Chenneville et al. (2010).

Goodness-of-Fit Ethical Framework

Fisher (2003, 2017) proposed that assent/consent processes for children should strive for "goodness-of-fit" between the child's decisional capacity and the nature of the research study. The argument in favour of this approach rests on the belief that allowing children the right to choose whether to participate in research study based solely on legal status denies them the right to exercise autonomy and agency (Fisher, 1999). Fisher (2003) articulates several reasons as to why children should have the final say with regard to participation in research including (1) the benefits and risks of participating in any given study are weighed by the Institutional

Review Board (IRB); (2) parents/guardians have the opportunity to make an informed decision regarding their child's participation after they have considered the risks & benefits, and (3) children's rights to autonomy are preserved when they are allowed to decide whether or not they want to participate in a research study. Researchers using the goodness-of-fit framework ensure the assent process meets the developmental level and decisional capacity of the child by: (1) providing children with educational information on research procedures and how they will be protected from harm prior to the assent process (Bruzzese & Fisher, 2003), (2) using age appropriate language and presentation methods (e.g. pictures) to explain the research procedures including benefits and risks (Fisher, 2003); (3) reassuring children they will not face any penalty should they choose not to give their assent (Fisher, 2003; Walker, 2002). Working in this way allows children to exercise their agency and meets the ethical requirement of respect for persons.

Protection-Autonomy Model

This model encourages researchers to assess the decisional capacity of children as some minors may be competent to not only give their assent, but consent to participate in a research study. Chenneville et al. (2010) recommend using the protection-autonomy decisional model to determine if a minor, defined as someone who is below the legal age of majority, is competent to give informed consent. This model asks researchers to consider the child's right to autonomy versus the need for protection (see Sturman, 2005 for a review of standardized assessment tools for assessment of competency). It is, however, important to remember that the right to give consent is typically determined by national laws and regulations. This means that even if a child is deemed competent to give informed consent, it may not be valid, and parental consent will still be needed.

Recommendations for Music Therapy Research with Children

In music therapy research, all actions concerning children must prioritize their best interests as a primary consideration, reflecting strong legal obligations to protect their rights while respecting their decisional capacity. As noted by Chenneville (2023), there are competing interests and views when determining if children are vulnerable and in need of protection, or if they are autonomous and capable of making informed decisions when it comes to research participation. These views will determine how much weight will be given to a child's decision to participate in a research study. Music therapists are encouraged to consider the legal and ethical requirements when balancing the "need for protection" versus the requirement for autonomy when inviting children to participate in a research study. The question to consider is whether a child's assent or refusal to participate in a music therapy research study should outweigh their parents'/guardian's consent or refusal. The two models described above (Fisher's goodness-of-fit & Chenneville et al.'s autonomy model) offer music therapists guidance on how best to involve children in research.

Children should be recognized as active participants in the research process, with consideration given to their cognitive ability to make informed decisions. Their willingness or concerns regarding participation in a research study should be weighed equally alongside those of their parents or guardians before determining their inclusion. To support ethical research practices, the following guidelines are proposed to help music therapists uphold the principles of autonomy, beneficence, and justice.

- Assess decisional capacity using the available tools to determine if a child can make an informed decision regarding research participation.
- Create age-appropriate materials that explain the research study's purpose, method, length of involvement, risks, and benefits using language that matches the child's cognitive abilities. Visual aids should be used to help a child understand all aspects of the study.
- Make sure the child understands they can withdraw from the study at any time. Reinforce the fact that there will not be any penalties or punishment should they choose to withdraw.
- Respect the child's autonomy. Music therapy researchers should work with parents so that a child's wish to participate, refuse to participate, or withdraw from a study is heard and respected. Encourage children to voice any concerns they may have regarding a particular research study.

(*continued*)

(continued)

- Seek assent from a child before enrolling them in a research study. Weigh their decisional capacity, especially when high, against parental/guardian concerns. Work with parents/guardians as necessary to ensure the child's voice is heard and respected.
- Children should be active participants in any research study involving them. Those with higher decisional capacity should have a meaningful say in their participation per Articles 12 and 13 of the UNCRC.
- Follow national and local laws/regulations regarding assent/consent procedures for a child's participation in research. Help children understand the legal requirements for parent/guardian consent, even if they have a high level of decisional capacity.
- Minimize risks to children who agree to participate in a research study. Take into consideration unintended consequences of participation (e.g. re-traumatization). Create a supportive environment to minimize risk and answer questions as they arise.
- Keep detailed documentation outlining the assent/consent process that was followed. Record how decisional capacity was assessed and decisions made to balance the right to autonomy and protection. Make note of a parent's/guardian's refusal to accept the child's decision to participate, refuse to participate, or withdraw from a research study and share that information with the research team.

References

Applebaum, P. S. (2007). Assessment of patients' competence to consent for treatment. *The New England Journal of Medicine, 357*(18), 1834–1840. https://doi.org/10.1056/NEJMcp74045

Bruzzese, J. B., & Fisher, C. B. (2003). Assessing and enhancing the research consent capacity of children and youth. *Applied Developmental Science, 7*, 13–26.

Chakraborty, K., Nansen, B., Gibbs, L., & MacDougall, C. (2012). Ethical negotiations: Committees, methods and research with children. *The International Journal of Children's Rights, 20*(4), 541–553. https://doi.org/10.1163/157181812x634472

Chenneville, T. (2023, December 3–6). *Research with minors: Balancing autonomy and protection* [Conference session]. 2023 PRIM&R Annual Conference, Washington, DC, United States.

Chenneville, T., Sibille, K., & Bendell-Estroff, D. (2010). Decisional capacity among minors with HIV: A model for balancing autonomy rights with the need for protection. *Ethics and Behavior, 20*(2), 83–94.

Crane, S., & Broome, M. E. (2017). Understanding ethical issues of research participation from the perspective of participating children and adolescents: A systematic review. *Worldviews on Evidence-Based Nursing, 14*(3), 200–209.

Fisher, C. B. (1999). Relational ethics and research with vulnerable populations. In *Reports on research involving persons with mental disorders that may affect decision-making capacity, Vol.* II, 29–49.

Fisher, C. B. (2003). A goodness-of-fit ethic for child assent to nonbeneficial research. *AJOB Research, 3*(4), 27–28.

Fisher, C. B. (2017). *Decoding the ethics code: A practical guide for psychologists* (4th ed.). Sage Publications.

Grisso, T., & Applebaum, P. S. (1998). *Assessing competence to consent to treatment: A guide for physicians and other health professionals.* Oxford University Press.

Hein, I. M., De Vries, M. C., Troost, P. W., Meynen, G., Van Doudoever, J. B., & Lindauer, R. J. L. (2015). Informed consent instead of assent is appropriate in children from the age of twelve: Policy implications for new findings on children's competence to consent to clinical research. *BMC Medical Ethics, 16*(1), 76. https://doi.org/10.1186/s12910-015-0067-z

Krappmann, L. (2010). The weight of the child's view (Article 12 of the Convention on the Rights of the Child). *International Journal of Children's Rights, 18*(4), 501–513.

Mastroianni, A. C., Faden, R., & Federman, D. (Eds.). (1994). *Institute of medicine (US) committee on ethical and legal issues relating to the inclusion of women in clinical studies.* National Academies Press. https://www.ncbi.nlm.nih.gov/books/NBK236544/

Merriam-Webster. (n.d.). Autonomy. In Merriam-Webster.com dictionary. Retrieved August 13, 2024, from https://www.merriam-webster.com/dictionary/autonomy

Miles, S. H. (2004). *The Hippocratic oath and the ethics of medicine.* Oxford University Press.

National Commission for the Protection of Human Subjects of Biomedical and Behavioral Research. (1979). *The Belmont report: Ethical principles and guidelines for the protection of human subjects of research.* U.S. Department of Health, Education, and Welfare. https://www.hhs.gov/ohrp/regulations-and-policy/belmont-report/index.html

Pieper, L., & Thomson, C. J. H. (2013). Justice in human research ethics. A conceptual and practice guide. *Monash Bioethics Review, 31*(1), 91–116.

Powell, M. A., & Smith, A. S. (2009). Children's participation rights in research. *Childhood, 16*(1), 124–142. https://doi.org/10.1177/0907566208101694

Pratt, B., Wild, V., Barasa, E., Kamuya, D., Gilson, L., Hendl, T., & Molyneux, S. (2020). Justice: A key consideration in health policy and systems research ethics. *BMJ Global Health, 5*, e001942. https://doi.org/10.1136/bmjgh-2019-001942

Regulation (EU) 2016/679. (2016, April 27). Regulation (EU) 2016/679 of the European Parliament and of the Council of 27 April 2016 on the protection of natural persons with regard to the processing of personal data and on the free movement of such data, and repealing Directive 95/46/EC (General Data Protection Regulation). *Official Journal of the European Union, L 119*, 1–88. https://eur-lex.europa.eu/eli/reg/2016/679/ojWikipedia+2Academia Stack Exchange+2

Roth, L. H., Meisel, A., & Lidz, C. W. (1977). Test of competency to consent to treatment. *American Journal of Psychiatry, 124*, 279–284.

Sinclair, R. (2004). Participation in practice: Making it meaningful, effective, and sustainable. *Children & Society, 18*, 106–118.

Sturman, E. D. (2005). The capacity to consent to treatment and research: A review of standardized assessment tools. *Clinical Psychology Review, 25*(7), 954–974.

UN Committee on the Rights of the Child (UNCRC). (2013). *General comment No. 14 on the right of the child to have his or her best interests taken as a primary consideration (art. 3, para. 1)*. CRC/C/GC/14. Retrieved from https://www2.ohchr.org/english/bodies/crc/docs/gc/crc_c_gc_14_eng.pdf

Walker, M. (2002). Autonomy, beneficence, and justice in the wider context. *Ethics and Behavior, 12*, 291–293.

West, D. (1998). Radiation experiments on children at the Fernald and Wrentham schools: Lessons for human subject research. *Accountability in Research: Policies & Quality Assurance, 6*(1/2), 103–125.

World Health Organization. (n.d.). *Mental health*. World Health Organization. https://www.who.int/health-topics/mental-health#tab=tab_1

World Medical Association. (2013). *WMA declaration of Helsinki—Ethical principles for medical research involving human subjects.*

CHAPTER 9

Concluding Thoughts

I used music a lot during difficult times.
—Participant in Krüger et al., *2024*, p. 9

As we have argued in this book, music therapy creates arenas for advancing children's rights. By illuminating these rights, societies can unlock innovative pathways to address children's needs, providing children with platforms for self-expression, access to therapeutic support, and mechanisms to safeguard their mental, emotional, and social well-being. To sum up, we will highlight six aspects of a child-centred music therapy approach.

Firstly, we argue that child-centred music therapy is deeply connected to the historical use of music for healing and emotional well-being, traditions that span ancient civilizations and diverse cultures. Modern frameworks, such as the United Nations Convention on the Rights of the Child (UNCRC), emphasize the protection and promotion of children's rights, ensuring that they have access to education, healthcare, and freedom from exploitation and abuse. They advocate for children's participation in decisions that affect them, upholding their right to be heard and respected. As we have argued, music therapy plays a significant role in advancing these rights by providing children with opportunities to express themselves, access therapeutic support, and safeguard their mental, emotional health and social. Raising awareness about children's rights is not merely an act of advocacy; it creates possibilities and mobilizes resources for change.

V. Krüger, K. M. Murphy, *Child-Centred Music Therapy*,
https://doi.org/10.1007/978-3-031-85724-9_9

Secondly, we emphasize that child-centred music therapy aligns with the principle of the *best interests of the child* (BID) by prioritizing children's unique needs, voices, and developmental goals. When professionals tailor interventions to the child's circumstances and aspirations, music therapy becomes a dynamic tool for personal growth and resilience. In this regard, listening to children is not optional but fundamental. Children's voices must inform the BID process, ensuring their active participation shapes decisions about their care and well-being. Music therapy techniques, such as songwriting and improvisation, provide children with arenas for communication and participation, which can help professionals better understand children's perspectives. Collaborative approaches and power-balancing strategies through music therapy have the potential to amplify children's voices while fostering inclusion among all stakeholders.

Thirdly, we underscore that child-centred music therapy involves critical reflection on roles and practices, challenging paternalistic assumptions that often silence children's voices. By incorporating culturally responsive, strength-based, and child-centred approaches—such as Resource-Oriented Music Therapy (ROMT) (Rolvsjord, 2010) and Community Music Therapy (CoMT) (Stige & Aarø, 2012)—practitioners can empower children to actively shape their therapeutic experiences. Drawing on Vygotsky's sociocultural theory (1978) and Lave and Wenger's communities of practice (1991), music therapy acknowledges the role of social and cultural contexts in children's development. We have explored the intersection of music therapy, critical childhood studies (CCS), and social justice, emphasizing the importance of a critical, reflexive approach for professionals working with children and adolescents, highlighting the need for music therapists to understand both the ecological contexts of children's development and the broader social structures that shaped their experiences. As such CCS integrate research to examine childhood as a social and cultural construct, utilizing qualitative methodologies to explore the diverse experiences of children in various contexts. Following this, a post-human perspective challenges traditional views on childhood by emphasizing interconnectedness between humans and technologies. In the "best interests of the child," this expands care to include factors like environmental and technological influences.

Fourthly, in search for a child-centred music therapy, we highlight the importance of professional discretion in navigating the complex interplay between therapeutic practices and children's rights. Music therapists must thoughtfully consider each child's needs, rights, and preferences, ensuring interventions are effective, respectful, and empowering. This requires practitioners to actively *listen* to children, not only to enhance therapy's impact but also to advocate for systemic changes that prioritize children's holistic development. A child-centred approach emphasizes creating a safe space for self-expression and involves the child in decision-making.

Fifthly, as recommended by Abrahams et al. (2024), among others, standardized documentation of child-centred music therapy practices is necessary to enhance clarity and comparability. This approach would provide a consistent framework for documenting and evaluating various music therapy interventions. However, as we strongly have advocated for by writing this book, it is crucial that this standardization is done while balancing the rights of the child, particularly the right to be heard. Respecting the child's voice and ensuring their active participation in the therapeutic process is essential. For example, children can be involved in the design and formulation of documentation and assessment tools for music therapy, ensuring their voices are heard and their perspectives are incorporated into the process. Children can be engaged in collaborative discussions where they share their thoughts on what is helpful in therapy and how they might like to assess their progress. Creative methods such as drawing, music-making, or role-playing allow children to express themselves in ways that can inform the development of assessment tools.

Sixthly, to realize a child-centred music therapy there is a need for more participatory research that prioritizes children's perspectives, recognizing them as active contributors rather than passive subjects. Although there are examples in settings like alternative care and schools, research amplifying children's voices remains scarce in many other contexts involving children. Involving children in research enriches our understanding of their experiences and empowers them to influence matters that impact their lives. This approach highlights the value of genuinely engaging children in shaping knowledge and decisions.

In conclusion, we believe that when children are recognized as active participants, not passive recipients, their voices can meaningfully inform therapeutic practices, policymaking, and resource allocation. To ensure that children's participation is authentic and impactful, professionals—music therapists included—must commit to amplifying children's voices and embedding them at the centre of their work. By doing so, we can move towards more accountable, responsive, sustainable, and inclusive practices that genuinely serve the best interests of the child.

References

Abrahams, T., van de Ree, M., Hakvoort, L., Konijn, C., Otten, R., Popma, A., & Nijhof, K. (2024). Music therapy and adverse childhood experiences: A scoping review. *Nordic Journal of Music Therapy.* https://doi.org/10.1080/08098131.2024.2388885

Krüger, V., Lexander, H., Fyhn, T. & Klette-Bøhler, K. (2024). Musisk medborgerskap –musikkverksted som tilnærming i forebyggende arbeid for unge, en kvalitativ analyse av kommunalt ansattes erfaringer. *Fontene Forskning.* [Musical citizenship—music workshop as an approach in preventive work for young people, a qualitative analysis of municipal employees' experiences]. (Fontene Research).

Lave, J., & Wenger, E. (1991). *Situated learning: Legitimate peripheral participation.* Cambridge University Press.

Rolvsjord, R. (2010). *Resource-oriented music therapy in mental health care.* Barcelona Publishers.

Stige, B., & Aarø, L. E. (2012). *Invitation to community music therapy.* Routledge.

Vygotsky, L. (1978). *Mind in society: The development of higher psychological processes.* Harvard University Press.

Appendix

Guidelines for Implementing Music Therapy Using the Best Interest Determination Process (BID).

1. Focusing on Individual Needs and Circumstances of Each Child's

Contribution: Music therapists significantly enhance the BID process by personalizing engagement, facilitating emotional expression, and taking a holistic understanding of each child into consideration.

Suggestions for Action:

<u>Create Individualized Music Therapy Plans:</u> Develop personalized music therapy experiences based on each child's preferences, emotional state, and communication style. Involve children in the planning process to ensure their preferences are reflected.

<u>Conduct Regular Assessments:</u> Conduct informal assessments of children's emotional and social development during music therapy sessions, adjusting choice of music experiences and procedures for

(*continued*)

V. Krüger, K. M. Murphy, *Child-Centred Music Therapy*,
https://doi.org/10.1007/978-3-031-85724-9

(continued)
engagement based on ongoing observations. Documentation should include an accurate representation of the child's view. This means that their words are accurately recorded, and they are given the chance to clarify or correct any statements, ensuring their voice is genuinely reflected throughout the process.

Provide Alternative Communication Tools: Provide children with various instruments, technologies, and materials for expression during music therapy sessions, encouraging them to communicate feelings through music, art, or movement.

Establish Safe Spaces: Create a comfortable, non-judgmental environment for children to explore their emotions and thoughts.

2. Enhancing Connections and Interactions Among Stakeholders

Contribution: Music therapists should promote collaboration among families, community organizations, and teams involved in a child's care.

Suggestions for Action:

Involve Families in Therapy: Conduct family-centred music therapy sessions to explore family dynamics and gather insights from family members about the child's needs and preferences.

Facilitate Community Partnerships: Collaborate with local organizations to connect families with resources and support networks that align with the child's needs, such as educational and mental health services.

Organize Workshops: Host workshops for professionals from different fields (e.g., education, healthcare, social work) to educate them on the benefits of children's participation in music therapy. Provide examples of how music can be used within the context of a music therapy session, or in other contexts fostering collaborative care approaches.

(*continued*)

(continued)

Develop Cultural Competence Training: Integrate training programs that educate therapists and stakeholders on various cultural traditions and practices related to music, enhancing understanding and respect for diverse backgrounds.

3. Influencing Broader Systemic Factors

Contribution: Music therapists may be able to influence systemic factors and external environments that impact a child's well-being through policy advocacy and community engagement.

Suggestions for Action:

Engage in Policy Advocacy: Collaborate with child welfare organizations to advocate for the inclusion of music therapy in legislation related to children's mental health, wellness, and education.

Conduct and Publish Research: Actively participate in research initiatives that demonstrate the effectiveness of music therapy in supporting children's emotional and social needs, sharing findings with stakeholders and policymakers.

Raise Community Awareness: Organize community events and workshops to educate parents, educators, and service providers about the benefits of music therapy, fostering support for its inclusion in BID assessments.

Develop Comprehensive Resource Networks: Collaborate with various organizations to create resource directories that connect families with music therapy services and other supportive programs.

4. Influencing Societal Structures and National Policies

Contribution: Music therapists contribute to the BID process by influencing overarching societal structures, cultural norms, and national policies affecting child welfare.

(*continued*)

(continued)

Suggestions for Action:

Advocate for Legislative Inclusion: Work with national organizations to ensure music therapy is recognized in child welfare legislation, advocating for its integration into national health and education policies.

Participate in Public Awareness Campaigns: Engage in campaigns that promote mental health awareness and the benefits of creative arts therapies, helping to destigmatize mental health issues and encourage families to seek services. In the case of including participants, protecting them from privacy intrusions is crucial, particularly with the increased use of social media.

Facilitate National and International Collaboration: Create forums for professionals from various disciplines to collaborate on developing integrated care models that prioritize children's best interests.

Contribute to Best Practice Guidelines: Participate in the development of best practice guidelines that incorporate music therapy into child welfare practices at the national level.

5. Recognizing Developmental Stages and Temporal Aspects

Contribution: Music therapists recognize the importance of time and the impact of developmental stages on a child's well-being. Music therapists should consider opportunities that provide services to children beyond the age of 18 to ensure that the therapeutic benefits continue to support the best interests of young adults as they transition into adulthood.

Suggestions for Action:

Tailor Interventions to Developmental Stages: Design therapy approaches that align with each child's developmental milestones, adjusting methods for different age groups to meet their unique needs.

(*continued*)

(continued)

Avoid Short-Term Solutions

Long-term well-being of the child is essential. While short-term solutions may offer immediate relief, they can undermine sustainable growth and development. Music therapists develop an approach that focuses on fostering resilience, enhancing relational connections, and promoting self-expression to ensure lasting positive outcomes that align with the child's best interests.

Provide Support During Transitions: Offer targeted music therapy support during significant life transitions, helping children navigate changes in their environment or family dynamics.

Implement Long-Term Engagement Strategies: Encourage ongoing music therapy engagement to promote resilience, emotional regulation, and social skills, assessing progress and adapting interventions as necessary.

Evaluate and Refine Practices: Conduct longitudinal studies to evaluate the effectiveness of music therapy in supporting children's developmental trajectories, sharing results to refine and improve practices.

References

Aalborg University. (n.d.). *Music therapy research – IMTAC*. https://www.communication.aau.dk/research/music-therapy-research/imtac#f6cdb6b6-a870-4fc7-a1e0-f62d69c216c0

Abrahams, T., van de Ree, M., Hakvoort, L., Konijn, C., Otten, R., Popma, A., & Nijhof, K. (2024). Music therapy and adverse childhood experiences: A scoping review. *Nordic Journal of Music Therapy*. https://doi.org/10.1080/08098131.2024.2388885

Aigen, K. (2005). *Music-centered music therapy*. Barcelona Publishers.

Ainscow, M. (2020). Promoting inclusion and equity in education: Lessons from international experiences. *Nordic Journal of Studies in Educational Policy, 6*(1), 7–16. https://doi.org/10.1080/20020317.2020.1729587

Aitchison, K. A., & Skewes McFerran, K. (2022). Six adolescents' lived experiences of resource-oriented music therapy assessment in a community-based mental health day program. *Arts in Psychotherapy, 81*, 101991. https://doi.org/10.1016/j.aip.2022.101991

Albornoz, Y. (2011). The effects of group improvisational music therapy on depression in young people and adults with substance abuse: A randomized controlled trial. *Nordic Journal of Music Therapy, 20*(3), 208–224. https://doi.org/10.1080/08098131.2010.522717

Alvarez, T. T. (2012). Beats, rhymes, and life. Rap therapy in an urban setting. In S. Hadley & G. Yancy (Eds.), *Therapeutic uses of rap and hip-hop* (pp. 117–128). Routledge.

V. Krüger, K. M. Murphy, *Child-Centred Music Therapy*,
https://doi.org/10.1007/978-3-031-85724-9

Andersen, T. (1987). The reflecting team: Dialogue and meta-dialogue in clinical work. *Family Process, 26*(4), 415–428. https://doi.org/10.1111/j.1545-5300.1987.00415.x

Ansdell, G. (2002). Community music therapy & the winds of change. *Voices: A World Forum for Music Therapy, 2*(2), 1–46. https://doi.org/10.15845/voices.v2i2.83

Applebaum, P. S. (2007). Assessment of patients' competence to consent for treatment. *The New England Journal of Medicine, 357*(18), 1834–1840. https://doi.org/10.1056/NEJMcp74045

Archard, D., & Skivenes, M. (2009). Balancing a child's best interests and the child's views. *International Journal of Children's Rights, 17*(1), 1–21.

Arendt, H. (1951). *The origins of totalitarianism*. Harcourt Brace.

Aristotle. (2015). *Politics* (C. D. C. Reeve, Trans.). Hackett Publishing Company.

Arnon, S., Epstein, S., Ghetti, C., Bauer-Rusek, S., Taitelbaum-Swead, R., & Yakobson, D. (2022). Music therapy intervention in an open bay neonatal intensive care unit room is associated with less noise and higher signal to noise ratios: A case-control study. *Children, 9*, 1187. https://doi.org/10.3390/children9081187

Arnstein, S. R. (1969). A ladder of citizen participation. *Journal of the American Planning Association, 35*(4), 216–224.

Austin, D. (2007). Lifesongs: Music therapy with adolescents in foster care. In V. Camilleri (Ed.), *Healing the inner-city child: Creative arts therapy with at-risk youth* (pp. 92–103). Jessica Kingsley Publishers.

Ayson, C. (2008). Child-parent wellbeing in a paediatric ward: The role of music therapy in supporting children and their parents facing the challenge of hospitalisation. *Voices: A World Forum for Music Therapy, 8*(1). https://doi.org/10.15845/voices.v8i1.449

Bağli, E., Küçükoğlu, S., & Soylu, H. (2024). The effect of lullabies and classical music on preterm neonates' cerebral oxygenation, vital signs, and comfort during orogastric tube feeding: A randomized controlled trial. *Biological Research for Nursing, 26*(2), 181–191. https://doi.org/10.1177/10998004231202404

Baines, S. (2013). Music therapy as an anti-oppressive practice. *The Arts in Psychotherapy, 40*(1), 1–5. https://doi.org/10.1016/j.aip.2012.09.003

Baker, F. A. (2013). An investigation of the sociocultural factors impacting on the therapeutic songwriting process. *Nordic Journal of Music Therapy, 23*(2), 123–151. https://doi.org/10.1080/08098131.2013.783094

Baker, F., & Jones, C. (2006). The effect of music therapy services on classroom behaviours of newly arrived refugee students in Australia: A pilot study. *Emotional and Behavioural Difficulties, 11*(4), 249–260. https://doi.org/10.1080/13632750601022170

Baker, F. A., Jeanneret, N., & Clarkson, A. (2018). Contextual factors and wellbeing outcomes: Ethnographic analysis of an artist-led group songwriting program with young people. *Psychology of Music, 46*(2), 266–280. https://doi.org/10.1177/0305735617709520

Band, J. P. (2019). Guided imagery and music with children and young people. In D. E. Grocke (Ed.), *Guided imagery and music: The Bonny method and beyond* (pp. 79–96). Barcelona Publishers.

Barnevernloven (Child welfare act), Section 1–3. https://lovdata.no/dokument/NL/lov/1992-07-17-100

Baron, A. (2017). Working with families in the acute pediatric medical setting. In S. L. Jacobsen & G. Thompson (Eds.), *Music therapy with families* (pp. 45–71). Jessica Kingsley Publishers.

Bates, D. (2014). Music therapy ethics "2.0": Preventing user error in technology. *Music Therapy Perspectives, 32*(2), 136–141. https://doi.org/10.1093/mtp/miu030

Bath, H. (2015). The three pillars of trauma-wise care: Healing in the other 23 hours. *Reclaiming Children and Youth, 23*(4), 44–46.

Bauer, A., Stevens, M., Purtscheller, D., Knapp, M., Fonagy, P., Evans-Lacko, S., & Paul, J. (2021). Mobilising social support to improve mental health for children and adolescents: A systematic review using principles of realist synthesis. *PLoS One, 16*(5), e0251750. https://doi.org/10.1371/journal.pone.0251750

Beckmann, H. B. (2013). Music, adolescents and health: Narratives about how young people use music as a health resource in daily life. In *Musical life stories: Narratives on health musicking* (Vol. 6). Centre for Music and Health Publication Series, NMH-publikasjoner

Beer, L. E., & Lee, K. (2017). Music therapy and procedural support: Defining and identifying areas of practice. *Music and Medicine, 9*(4), 262–267.

Bell, S. A. (2016). *A music therapist's self-reflection on her aboriginal heritage: A heuristic self-inquiry* (Master's thesis). Concordia University, Montreal.

Bieleninik, Ł., & Ghetti, C. (2019). Music therapy for preterm infants and their parents: A path forward for research in Poland. *Roczniki Psychologiczne/Annals of Psychology, 22*(2), 135–150. https://doi.org/10.18290/rpsych.2019.22.2-3

Birch, J., & Thompson, G. (2023). Exploring music therapy research in preschool settings that include children with disabilities: A scoping review. *The Journal of Music Therapy, 60*(1), 64–97. https://doi.org/10.1093/jmt/thac015

Blacking, J. (1978). *How musical is man?* University of Washington Press.

Blaxter, M. (2010). *Health*. Polity.

Bolger, L. (2013). Music therapy and international development in action and reflection: A case study of a women's music group in rural Bangladesh. *Australian Journal of Music Therapy, 23*, 22–38.

Bonde, L. O. (2020). Music and health promotion in Danish/Nordic hospitals—who and how? An essay. In L. O. Bonde & K. Johansson (Eds.), *Music in paediatric hospitals—Nordic perspectives* (pp. 149–169). Series from Centre for Research in Music and Health (CREMAH).

British Columbia Ministry of Children and Family Development. (n.d.). *Agreements with young adults (AYA)*. Government of British Columbia. Retrieved December 16, 2024, from https://www2.gov.bc.ca/gov/content/family-social-supports/youth-and-family-services/teens-in-foster-care/agreements-with-young-adults

Brodie, E., Cowling, E., Nissen, N., Paine, A., Jochum, V., & Warburton, D. (2009). *Understanding participation: A literature review*. NCVO.

Bronfenbrenner, U. (1979). *The ecology of human development: Experiments by nature and design*. Harvard University Press.

Brown, J. M. (2002). Towards a culturally centered music therapy practice. *Voices: A World Forum for Music Therapy, 2*(1). https://doi.org/10.15845/voices.v2i1.72

Bruscia, K. E. (1998). *The dynamics of music psychotherapy*. Barcelona Publishers.

Bruscia, K. E. (2014). *Defining music therapy* (3rd ed.). Barcelona Publishers.

Bruscia, K. E. (2015). *Reflexivity in music therapy: An anthology*. Barcelona Publishers.

Bruzzese, J. B., & Fisher, C. B. (2003). Assessing and enhancing the research consent capacity of children and youth. *Applied Developmental Science, 7*, 13–26.

Burns, D. S., Robb, S. L., & Haase, J. E. (2009). Exploring the feasibility of a therapeutic music video intervention in adolescents and young adults during stem-cell transplantation. *Cancer Nursing, 32*(5), E8–E16. https://doi.org/10.1097/NCC.0b013e3181a4802c

Burroughs, M. D., & Tollefsen, D. (2016). Learning to listen: Epistemic injustice and the child. *Episteme, 13*(3), 359–377.

Buzzi, F., Yahya, N. B., Gambazza, S., Binda, F., Galazzi, A., Ferrari, A., Crespan, S., Al-Atroushy, H. A., Cantoni, B. M., Laquintana, D., & Collaborative Group. (2022). Use of musical intervention in the pediatric intensive care unit of a developing country: A pilot pre–post study. *Children, 9*, 455. https://doi.org/10.3390/children9040455

Calabro, J., & Grocke, D. E. (2017). Music therapy for infants with neonatal abstinence syndrome. *Music & Medicine, 9*(1), 37–44.

Caló, F., Steiner, A., Millar, S., & Teasdale, S. (2020). The impact of a community-based music intervention on the health and well-being of young people: A realist evaluation. *Health & Social Care in the Community, 28*(3), 988–997.

Carel, H., & Kidd, I. J. (2014). Epistemic injustice in healthcare: A philosophial analysis. *Medicine, Health Care and Philosophy, 17*, 529–540.

Carr, C., & Wigram, T. (2009). Music therapy with children and adolescents in mainstream schools: A systematic review. *British Journal of Music Therapy, 23*(1), 3–18. https://doi.org/10.1177/135945750902300102

Center for Disease Control. (2024, November 8). *Preterm birth*. https://www.cdc.gov/maternal-infant-health/preterm-birth/index.html

Center for Disease Control and Prevention (CDC). (2024a, August 20). *About children's mental health*. https://www.c.gov/children-mental-health/about/index.html

Center for Disease Control and Prevention (CDC). (2024b, October 8). *About adverse childhood experiences*. https://www.cdc.gov/aces/about/

Chakraborty, K., Nansen, B., Gibbs, L., & MacDougall, C. (2012). Ethical negotiations: Committees, methods and research with children. *The International Journal of Children's Rights, 20*(4), 541–553. https://doi.org/10.1163/157181812x634472

Chase, K. M. (2004). Therapy with gay and lesbian clients: Implications for music therapists. *Music Therapy Perspectives, 22*(1), 34–38. https://doi.org/10.1093/mtp/22.1.34

Chenneville, T. (2023, December 3–6). *Research with minors: Balancing autonomy and protection* [Conference session]. 2023 PRIM&R Annual Conference, Washington, DC, United States.

Chenneville, T., Sibille, K., & Bendell-Estroff, D. (2010). Decisional capacity among minors with HIV: A model for balancing autonomy rights with the need for protection. *Ethics and Behavior, 20*(2), 83–94.

Chetta, H. D. (1981). The effect of music and desensitization on preoperative anxiety in children. *Journal of Music Therapy, 18*(2), 74–87.

Children and Families Act 2014, c.6. https://www.legislation.gov.uk/ukpga/2014/6/contents/enacted

Children, Youth and Family Services Act. 2017. S.O. 2017, c. 14, Sched. 1. Retrieved from https://www.ontario.ca/laws/statute/17c14

Chong, H. J., & Kim, S. J. (2016). Education-oriented music therapy as an after-school program for students with emotional and behavioural problems. *The Arts in Psychotherapy, 37*(3), 190–196. https://doi.org/10.1016/j.aip.2010.03.004

Christenbury, K. R. (2017). I will follow you: The combined use of songwriting and art to promote healing in a child who has been traumatized. *Music Therapy Perspectives, 35*(1), 1–12. https://doi.org/10.1093/mtp/miv005

Civil Society Coalition Norway. (2019). *Alternative report to the UN Committee on the rights of persons with disabilities*. https://unge-funksjonshemmede.no/rapport-til-fn-funksjonshemmedes-rettigheter-brytes-i-norge/

Cobbett, S. (2016). Context and relationships: Using the systemic approach with music therapy in work with children, adolescents, and their families. *British Journal of Music Therapy, 30*(2), 65–73.

Colegrove, V., Havighurst, S. S., Kehoe, C. E., & Jacobsen, S. L. (2018). Pilot randomized controlled trial of tuning relationships with music: Intervention for parents with a trauma history and their adolescents. *Child Abuse & Neglect, 79*, 259–268. https://doi.org/10.1016/j.chiabu.2018.01.001

Committee on Environmental Health. (1997). Noise: A hazard for the fetus and newborn. *Pediatrics, 100*, 724–727.

Comte, R. (2016). Neo-colonialism in music therapy: A critical interpretive synthesis of the literature concerning music therapy practice with refugees. *Voices: A World Forum for Music Therapy, 16*(3). https://doi.org/10.15845/voices.v16i3.865

Cook-Cottone, C. P., Kane, L., & Anderson, L. (2019). *The elements of counseling children and adolescents.* Springer Publishing Company.

Costa-Giomi, E. (2004). Effects of three years of piano instruction on children's academic achievement, school performance, and self-esteem. *Psychology of Music, 32*(2), 139–152. https://doi.org/10.1177/0305735604032002004

Cotter, K. E., & Krüger, V. (in press). Music therapy and family systems theory. In B. Wheeler, A. Dos Santos, & M. Viega (Eds.), *Music therapy handbook.* Guildford Press.

Crane, S., & Broome, M. E. (2017). Understanding ethical issues of research participation from the perspective of participating children and adolescents: A systematic review. *Worldviews on Evidence-Based Nursing, 14*(3), 200–209.

Curtis, S., & Vaillancourt, G. (2012). The children's right to music project. *Voices: A World Forum for Music Therapy, 12*(3).

Davies, E., & Rosscornes, C. (2012). Setting up and developing music therapy at a children's centre, for pre-school children and their families and carers. In J. Tomlinson, P. Derrington, & A. Oldfield (Eds.), *Music therapy in schools: Working with children of all ages in mainstream and special education* (pp. 19–32). Jessica Kingsley Publishers.

DeBacker, J. (1993). Containment in music therapy. In M. H. Heal & T. Wigram (Eds.), *Music therapy in health and education* (pp. 93–39). Jessica Kingsley Publisher.

Del Olmo, M. J., Rodríguez, C., & Ruza, F. (2010). Music therapy in the PICU: 0- to 6-month-old babies. *Music and Medicine, 2*(3), 158–166.

Del Ormo, M. J., Tarrio, F. R., Garrido, C. R., & marina, P. C. (2015). The effects of a music therapy intervention in PICU as measured by the comfort behavior scale. *Music and Medicine, 7*(2), 20–24.

Deleuze, G. (1990). *The logic of sense* (M. Lester & C. Stivale, Trans.). Columbia University Press.

Deleuze, G., & Parnet, C. (2002). *Dialogues II* (H. Tomlinson & B. Habberjam, Trans.). Columbia University Press.

DeNora, T. (2007). Health and music in everyday life: A theory of practice. *Psyke & Logos, 28*, 271–287.

Derrington, P. (2019). "What's the WiFi code here?": Connecting with adolescents in music therapy. In K. McFerran, P. Derrington, & S. Saarikallio (Eds.), *Handbook of music, adolescents, and well-being* (pp. 165–175). Oxford University Press.

Devlin, K., Johnston, M., & Johnston, C. (2024). Making mistakes together: Therapy participant, parent, and therapist perspectives on music therapy in two different settings. *Music Therapy Perspectives, 42*(2), 129–138. https://doi.org/10.1093/mtp/miae007

Donley, J. (2020). Multicultural experiential learning in music therapy supervision. *Voices: A World Forum for Music Therapy, 20*(1), 1–2020. https://doi.org/10.15845/voices.v20i1.3005

Dorscheidt, J. H. H., & m, & Hein, I. M. (2018). Medical research involving children—Giving weight to children's views. *International Journal of Children's Rights, 26*, 93–116.

Dove, E. S., Avard, D., Black, L., & Knoppers, B. M. (2013). Emerging issues in paediatric health research consent forms in Canada: Working towards best practices. *BMC Medical Ethics, 14*(1), 14–25. https://doi.org/10.1186/1472-6939-14-5

Dovran, A., Winje, D., Arefjord, K., & Haugland, B. S. M. (2012). Traumatic events and posttraumatic reactions among children and adolescents in out-of-home placement: A 25-year systematic literature review. *Journal of Child and Adolescent Trauma, 5*(1), 6–32. https://doi.org/10.1080/19361521.2012.644654

Due, F. B., & Ghetti, C. (2018). Implementation of music therapy at a Norwegian children's hospital: A focused ethnographic study. *Voices: A World Forum for Music Therapy, 18*(2), 1–21.

Dun, B. (2013). Children with cancer. In J. Bradt (Ed.), *Guidelines for music therapy practice in pediatric care* (pp. 292–323). Barcelona Publishers.

Durkheim, È. (1951). *Suicide: A study in sociology* (J. A. Spaulding & G. Simpson, Trans.). The Free Press. (Original work published 1897).

Edwards, J. (2011). The use of music therapy to promote attachment between parents and infants. *The Arts in Psychotherapy, 38*(3), 190–195.

Edwards, J. (2023). Cultural humility in music therapy practice. In L. E. Beer & J. C. Birnbaum (Eds.), *Trauma-informed music therapy* (pp. 28–36). Routledge.

Edwards, J., & Kennelly, J. (2016). Music therapy for hospitalized children. In J. Edwards (Ed.), *The Oxford handbook of music therapy* (pp. 53–65). Oxford University Press. https://doi.org/10.1016/j.aip.2011.05.002

Einarsen, O. K., Krüger, V., Engebretsen, I. M. S., & Stige, B. (2024). Collaboration between social workers and music therapists in a child welfare context for unaccompanied refugee children: A focus group study. *Voices: A World Forum for Music Therapy, 24*(3) https://doi.org/10.15845/voices.v24i3.4071

Elefant, C. (2010). Unmasking hidden resources: Communication in children with severe developmental disabilities in music therapy. In V. Karkou (Ed.), *Arts therapies in schools: Research and practice* (pp. 243–258). Jessica Kingsley Publishers.

Enge, K. E. A., & Stige, B. (2022). Musical pathways to the peer community: A collective case study of refugee children's use of music therapy. *Nordic Journal of Music Therapy, 31*(1), 7–24. https://doi.org/10.1080/08098131.2021.1891130

Epp, E. (2007). Locating the autonomous voice: Self-expression in music-centered music therapy. *Voices: A World Forum for Music Therapy, 7*(1). https://doi.org/10.15845/voices.v7i1.463

Epstein, S., Elefant, C., Arnon, S., & Ghetti, C. (2023). Music therapy spanning from NICU to home: An interpretative phenomenological analysis of Israeli parents' experiences in the LongSTEP trial. *Nordic Journal of Music Therapy, 32*(5), 373–396. https://doi.org/10.1080/08098131.2023.2180773

Eriksen, M. H. (2017). Don't all mothers love their children? Deposited infants as animate objects in the Scandinavian iron age. *World Archaeology, 49*(3), 338–356. https://doi.org/10.1080/00438243.2017.1340189

European Union. (n.d.). *General data protection regulation (GDPR)*. Retrieved December 30, 2024, from https://gdpr-info.eu

Fairchild, R., & McFerran, K. S. (2019). "Music is everything": Using collaborative group songwriting as an arts-based method with children experiencing homelessness and family violence. *Nordic Journal of Music Therapy, 28*(2), 88–107. https://doi.org/10.1080/08098131.2018.1530189

Fairchild, R., & Mraz, M. (2018). "Everything changed when I got those drums": A collaborative case reflection. *Voices: A World Forum for Music Therapy, 18*(1), 1–13. https://doi.org/10.15845/voices.v18i1.957

Fairchild, R., & Sheridan, J. (2018). Strengthening bonds between children, young people, and their families after family violence. *Voices: A World Forum for Music Therapy, 18*(4), 1–13. https://doi.org/10.15845/voices.v18i4.2600

Fairchild, R., Thompson, G., & McFerran, K. S. (2017). Exploring the meaning of a performance in music therapy for children and their families experiencing homelessness and family violence. *Music Therapy Perspectives, 35*(1), 36–49. https://doi.org/10.1093/mtp/miw004

Falch-Eriksen, A., & Backe-Hansen, E. (2018). Child protection and human rights: A call for professional practice and policy. In A. Falch-Eriksen & E. Backe-Hansen (Eds.), *Human rights in child protection: Implications for professional practice* (pp. 1–15). Palgrave Macmillan.

Fancourt, D., & Finn, S. (2019). *What is the evidence on the role of the arts in improving health and wellbeing? A scoping review* (Health Evidence Network synthesis report, 6). World Health Organization Regional Office for Europe. https://www.euro.who.int/en/publications/abstracts/what-is-the-evidence-on-the-role-of-the-arts-in-improving-health-and-well-being-a-scoping-review-2019

Felitti, V. J., & Anda, R. F. (2010). The relationship of adverse childhood experiences to adult medical disease, psychiatric disorders, and sexual behavior:

Implications for healthcare. In R. Lanius & E. Vermette (Eds.), *The hidden epidemic: The impact of early life trauma on health and disease* (pp. 77–87). Cambridge University Press.

Felsenstein, R. (2013). From uprooting to replanting: On post-trauma group music therapy for pre-school children. *Nordic Journal of Music Therapy, 22*(1), 69–85. https://doi.org/10.1080/08098131.2012.667824

Finnish National Agency for Education. (2022). *National core curriculum for early childhood education and care.* https://www.oph.fi/sites/default/files/documents/Varhaiskasvatussuunnitelman%20perusteet%202022_EN_final_23%20.pdf

Fisher, C. B. (1999). Relational ethics and research with vulnerable populations. In *Reports on research involving persons with mental disorders that may affect decision-making capacity, Vol.* II, 29–49.

Fisher, C. B. (2003). A goodness-of-fit ethic for child assent to nonbeneficial research. *AJOB Research, 3*(4), 27–28.

Fisher, C. B. (2017). *Decoding the ethics code: A practical guide for psychologists* (4th ed.). Sage Publications.

Fisher, C. B., Arbeit, M. R., & Chenneville, T. (2017). Goodness-of-fit ethics for practice and research involving children and adolescents with HIV. In T. Chenneville (Ed.), *A clinical guide to pediatric HIV: Bridging the gaps between research and practice* (pp. 229–259). Springer International Publishing.

Fortin, J. (2006). Accommodating children's rights in a post-human rights act era. *The Modern Law Review, 69*(3), 299–326. https://www.jstor.org/stable/3699029

Foucault, M. (1982). The subject and power. *Critical Inquiry, 8*(4), 777–795. https://doi.org/10.1086/448181

Fricker, M. (2007). *Epistemic injustice. Power and the ethics of knowing.* Oxford University.

Gaden, T. S., Ghetti, C., Kvestad, I., & Gold, C. (2021a). The longSTEP approach: Theoretical framework and intervention protocol for using parent-driven infant-directed singing as resource-oriented music therapy. *Nordic Journal of Music Therapy, XX*(XX), 1–26. https://doi.org/10.1080/08098131.2021.1921014

Gaden, T. S., Ghetti, C., Kvestad, I., Bieleninik, Ł., Størksen Stordal, A., Assmus, J., Arnon, S., Elefant, C., Ettenberger, M., Lichtensztejn, M., Manger-snes, J., Janner Røed, C., Vederhus, B. J., & Gold, C. (2021b). Short-term music therapy for families with premature infants: The LongSTEP randomized trial. *Pediatrics.*

Gaden, T. S., Ghetti, C., Kvestad, I., Bieleninik, Ł., Stordal, A. S., Assmus, J., Arnon, S., Elefant, C., Epstein, S., Ettenberger, M., Lichtensztejn, M., Lindvall, M. W., Mangersnes, J., Røed, C. J., Vederhus, B. J., & Gold, C. (2022). Short-term Music Therapy for Families With Preterm Infants: A Randomized Trial.

Pediatrics, 149(2), e2021052797. https://doi.org/10.1542/peds.2021-052797

Geipel, J., Koenigb, J., Hillecke, T. K., Reschch, F., & Kaess, M. (2018). Music-based interventions to reduce internalizing symptoms in children and adolescents: A meta-analysis. *Journal of Affective Disorders, 225*, 647–656.

Gergen, K. (2009). *Relational being: Beyond self and community.* Oxford University Press.

Ghetti, C. M. (2012). Music therapy as procedural support for invasive medical procedures: Towards the development of music therapy theory. *Nordic Journal of Music Therapy, 2*(11), 3–35. https://doi.org/10.1080/08098131.2011.571278

Ghetti, C. M. (2013). Pediatric intensive care. In J. Bradt (Ed.), *Guidelines for music therapy practice in pediatric care* (pp. 152–204). Barcelona Publishers.

Ghetti, C. M. (2015). Maintaining the dialogue of influence: Developing music therapy theory in pace with practice and research. *Approaches: Music Therapy & Special Music Education, 7*(1), 30–37.

Ghetti, C. (2016). Performing a family of practices: Developments in community music therapy across international contexts. *Music Therapy Perspectives, 34*(2), 161–170. https://doi.org/10.1093/mtp/miv047

Ghetti, C., & Hannan, A. (2008). Pediatric intensive care unit. In D. Hanson-Abromeit & C. Colwell (Eds.), *Music therapy for pediatrics in hospital settings* (pp. 71–106). American Music Therapy Association.

Ghetti, C., & Walker, J. (2008). Hematology, oncology, and bone-marrow transplant. In D. Hanson-Abromeit & C. Colwell (Eds.), *Music therapy for pediatrics in hospital settings* (pp. 147–193). American Music Therapy Association.

Ghetti, C., Bieleninik, Ł., Hysing, M., Kvestad, I., Assmus, J., Romeo, R., Ettenberger, M., Arnon, S., Vederhus, B. J., Gaden, T. S., & Gold, C. (2019). Longitudinal study of music therapy's effectiveness for premature infants and their caregivers (LongSTEP): Protocol for an international randomized trial. *BMJ Open, 9*, e025062. https://doi.org/10.1136/bmjopen-2018-025062

Ghetti, C., Chen, X.-J., Brenner, A. K., Hakvoort, L. G., Lien, L., Fachner, J., & Gold, C. (2020). Music therapy for people with substance use disorders (Protocol). *Cochrane Database of Systematic Reviews, 2020*(10) Art. No.: CD012576. https://doi.org/10.1002/14651858.CD012576.pub2

Ghetti, C., Vederhus, B. J., Gaden, T. S., Brenner, A. K., Bieleninik, Ł., Kvestad, I., Assmus, J., & Gold, C. (2021). Longitudinal study of music therapy's effectiveness for premature infants and their caregivers (LongSTEP): Feasibility study with a Norwegian cohort. *Journal of Music Therapy, 58*(2), 201–240. https://doi.org/10.1093/jmt/thaa023

Ghetti, C. M., Gaden, T. S., Bieleninik, L., Kvestad, I., Assmus, J., Stordal, A. S., Aristizabal Sanchez, L. F., Arnon, S., Dulsrud, J., Elefant, C., Epstein, S., Ettenberger, M., Glosli, H., Konieczna-Nowak, L., Lichtensztejn, M., Lindvall,

M. W., Mangersnes, J., Murcia Fernández, L. D., Røed, C. J., Saá, G., van Roy, B., Vederhus, B. J., & Gold, C. (2023). Effect of music therapy on parent-infant bonding among infants born preterm: A randomized clinical trial. *JAMA Network Open, 6*(5), e2315750. https://doi.org/10.1001/jamanetworkopen.2023.15750

Giannelli, E., Gold, C., Bieleninik, Ł., Ghetti, C., & Gelo, O. C. G. (2019). Dialectical behaviour therapy and 12-step programmes for substance use disorder: A systematic review and meta-analysis. *Counselling and Psychotherapy Research, 00*, 1–12.

Giddens, A. (1984). *The constitution of society: Outline of the theory of structuration*. University of California Press.

Giddens, A. (1990). *The consequences of modernity*. Polity Press.

Gill, A., & Rickard, N. S. (2012). Non-musical benefits of school-based music education and training. In N. S. Rickard & K. McFerran (Eds.), *Lifelong engagement with music: Benefits for mental health and well-being* (pp. 57–72). Nova. https://doi.org/10.15845/voices.v23i1.3642

Gillett-Swan, J., Thelander, N., & Hanna, A. (2021). Setting the scene for children's rights and education: Understanding the aims of education. In J. Gillett-Swan & N. Thelander (Eds.), *Children's rights from international educational perspectives* (Transdisciplinary Perspectives in Educational Research) (Vol. 2). Springer. https://doi.org/10.1007/978-3-030-80861-7_1

Giordano, F., Zanchi, B., De Leonardis, F., Rutigliano, C., Esposito, F., Brienza, N., & Santoro, N. (2020). The influence of music therapy on preoperative anxiety in pediatric oncology patients undergoing invasive procedures. *The Arts in Psychotherapy*, 68. https://s443-doi-org.libdatabase.newpaltz.edu/10.1016/j.aip.2020.101649

Gold, C., Voracek, M., & Wigram, T. (2004). Effects of music therapy for children and adolescents with psychopathology: A meta-analysis. *Journal of Child Psychology and Psychiatry, 45*(6), 1054–1059.

Gold, C., Saarikallio, S., Crooke, A. H. D., & McFerran, K. S. (2017). Group music therapy as a preventive intervention for young people at risk: A cluster-randomized trial. *Journal of Music Therapy, 54*(2), 133–160.

Goldbeck, L., & Ellerkamp, T. (2012). A randomized controlled trial of multimodal music therapy for children with anxiety disorders. *Journal of Music Therapy, 49*(4), 395–413.

Gonzalez, P. J. (2011). The impact of music therapists' music cultures on the development of their professional frameworks. *Qualitative Inquiries in Music Therapy, 6*, 1–33.

Goodman, K. D. (2011). *Music therapy education and training: From theory to practice*. Charles C. Thomas Publisher.

Gottfried, T., Thompson, G., Elefant, C., & Gold, C. (2018). Reliability of the Music in Everyday Life (MEL) scale: A parent-report assessment for children on the autism spectrum. *Journal of Music Therapy, 55*, 133–155. https://doi.org/10.1093/jmt/thy002

Gouk, P. (2017). Introduction. In P. Gouk (Ed.), *Musical healing in cultural contexts* (pp. 1–25). Routledge.

Gravestock, J. (2021). *Music therapy in adoption and trauma: Therapy that makes a difference after placement.* Jessica Kingsley Publishers.

Grisso, T., & Applebaum, P. S. (1998). *Assessing competence to consent to treatment: A guide for physicians and other health professionals.* Oxford University Press.

Guerriero, A., & Blank, C. A. (2018). Music therapy in a parent-child reunification program: Benefits and challenges of implementation. *Voices: A World Forum for Music Therapy, 18*(4, special issue: Music therapy and child welfare).

Hadley, S. (Ed.). (2006). *Feminist perspectives in music therapy.* Barcelona Publishers.

Hadley, S., & Norris, M. S. (2016). Musical multicultural competency in music therapy: The first step. *Music Therapy Perspectives, 34*(2), 129–137.

Hadley, S., & Yancy, G. (Eds.). (2012). *Therapeutic Uses of Rap and Hip-Hop.* Routledge.

Haering, S. I. (2022). *The impact of music therapy on children in a multicultural elementary school* (1st ed.). Springer Fachmedien Wiesbaden. https://doi.org/10.1007/978-3-658-39330-4

Hailes, H. P., Yu, R., Danese, A., & Fazel, S. (2019). Long-term outcomes of childhood sexual abuse: An umbrella review. *The Lancet Psychiatry, 6*(10), 830–839. https://doi.org/10.1016/S2215-0366(19)30286-X

Hakomäki, H. (2012). Storycomposing as a method in music therapy. A collaborative experiment with a young co-researcher. In G. Trondalen & K. Stensæth (Eds.), *Barn, musikk, helse* (Vol. 3). Series from Centre for Research in Music and Health (CREMAH).

Hardirce, J. (2014). An overview of research ethics and learning from the past. *British Journal of Nursing, 23*(9), 483–486.

Hargrave, T. D., & Pfitzer, F. (2003). *The new contextual therapy: Guiding the power of give and take.* Brunner-Routledge.

Haslbeck, F. B. (2013). Creative music therapy with premature infants: An analysis of video footage. *Nordic Journal of Music Therapy, 23*(1), 5–31. https://doi.org/10.1080/08098131.2013.780091

Hayes, T. (2016). Music therapy in the context of the special school. In J. Edwards (Ed.), *The Oxford handbook of music therapy* (pp. 176–185). Oxford University Press.

Hegde, S. (2019). Neurologic music therapy targeting cognitive and affective functions. In M. H. Thaut & D. A. Hodges (Eds.), *The Oxford handbook of music and the brain.* Oxford University Press. https://doi.org/10.1093/oxfordhb/9780198804123.013.29

Heiderscheit, A., & Murphy, K. M. (2021). Trauma-informed care in music therapy: Principles, guidelines, and a clinical case illustration. *Music Therapy Perspectives, 39*(2), 142–151.

Hein, I. M., De Vries, M. C., Troost, P. W., Meynen, G., Van Doudoever, J. B., & Lindauer, R. J. L. (2015). Informed consent instead of assent is appropriate in children from the age of twelve: Policy implications for new findings on children's competence to consent to clinical research. *BMC Medical Ethics, 16*(1), 76. https://doi.org/10.1186/s12910-015-0067-z

Helander, S., Gattino, G. S., & Baumann, E. (2020). How music therapy is perceived in a pediatric outpatient chemotherapy unit in a Peruvian hospital: Report of an experience. *Revista Brasileira de Musicoterapia, 22*(29), 36–52. https://doi.org/10.51914/brjmt.29.2020.387

Helle-Valle, A. (2016). *How do we understand children's restlessness? A cooperative and reflexive exploration of children's restlessness as a bioecological phenomenon* (Doctoral dissertation). University of Bergen.

Helle-Valle, A., Binder, P.-E., Anderssen, N., & Stige, B. (2017). Is restlessness best understood as a process? Reflecting on four boys' restlessness during music therapy in kindergarten. *International Journal of Qualitative Studies on Health and Well-Being, 12*(supl), 1298266–1298215. https://doi.org/10.1080/17482631.2017.1298266

Hense, C., & McFerran, K. S. (2017). Promoting young people's musical identities to facilitate recovery from mental illness. *Journal of Youth Studies, 20*(8), 997–1012. https://doi.org/10.1080/13676261.2017.1287882

Hense, C., McFerran, K. S., Killackey, E., & McGorry, P. D. (2015). How can research practice promote young people's recovery from mental illness: A critical look at the Australian context. *Youth Voice Journal.* https://doi.org/10.1093/mtp/miz014

Heynen, E., Bruls, V., van Goor, S., Pat-El, R., Schoot, T., & van Hooren, S. (2022). A music therapy intervention for refugee children and adolescents in schools: A process evaluation using a mixed method design. *Children, 9*(10), 1434. https://doi.org/10.3390/children9101434

Hilliard, R. E. (2003). Music therapy in pediatric palliative care: Complementing the interdisciplinary approach. *Journal of Palliative Care, 19*, 127–132.

Hindle, S. (2000). *The state and social change in early modern England.* Palgrave Macmillan.

Houston, S. (2017). Towards a critical ecology of child development in social work: Aligning the theories of Bronfenbrenner and Bourdieu. *Families, Relationships and Societies, 6*(1), 53–69. https://doi.org/10.1332/204674315X14281321359847

Hoy, N., Lynch, S. J., Waszczuk, M. A., Reppermund, S., & Mewton, L. (2023). Transdiagnostic biomarkers of mental illness across the lifespan: A systematic review examining the genetic and neural correlates of latent transdiagnostic dimensions of psychopathology in the general population. *Neuroscience and Biobehavioral Reviews, 155*, 105431. https://doi.org/10.1016/j.neubiorev.2023.105431

Hunt, A. (1990). Rights and social movements: Counter-hegemonic strategies. *Journal of Law and Society, 17*(3), 309–328.

Hunt, M. (2005). Action research and music therapy: Group music therapy with young refugees in a school community. *Voices: A World Forum for Music Therapy, 5*(2). https://doi.org/10.15845/voices.v5i2.223

Hussey, D. L., Reed, A. M., Laymann, D. L., & Pasiali, V. (2007). Music therapy and complex trauma: A protocol for developing social reciprocity. *Residential Treatment for Children & Youth, 24*(1–2), 111–129. https://doi.org/10.1300/J007v24n01_07

Institute for Patient- and Family-Centered Care. (n.d.). *Patient-and family-cantered care*. https://www.ipfcc.org/about/pfcc.html

International Music Council. (n.d.). *Home*. International Music Council. https://imc-cim.org/

Iyendo, T. O., Makanjuola, O. B., & Ojo, T. M. (2024). Effect of audio-visual-based art and music therapy in reducing adolescents' post-traumatic stress disorder. *Journal of Adolescent Health, 74*(2), 283–291. https://doi.org/10.1016/j.jadohealth.2023.07.008

Jackson, N. (2018). Therapeutic lessons with a girl with Down syndrome. In A. Heiderscheit & N. Jackson (Eds.), *Introduction to music therapy practice* (pp. 33–39). Barcelona Publishers.

Jacobsen, S. L. (2019). Musikterapi i udredning og behandling af udsatte børn og familier. *Tidsskriftet Norges Barnevern, 96*(1–2), 56–68.

Jacobsen, S. L., & McKinney, C. H. (2015). A music therapy tool for assessing parent–child interaction in cases of emotional neglect. *Journal of Child and Family Studies, 24*(7), 2164–2173. https://doi.org/10.1007/s10826-014-0022-6

Jacobsen, S. L., & Thompson, G. (2017). *Music therapy with families: Therapeutic approaches and theoretical perspectives*. Jessica Kingsley Publishers.

Jebb, E. (1924). *Declaration of the rights of the child*. League of Nations.

Jensen, F. P., Križ, K., & Skivenes, M. (2022, July 11). *Structuring practice for children's participation: Report I for the participation project: Mapping and evaluating organizational guidelines*. Centre for Research on Discretion and Paternalism, University of Bergen.

Johanson, K., & Bonde, L. O. (Eds.). (n.d.). *Music in paediatric hospitals—Nordic perspectives*. Norwegian Academy of Music.

Johansson, K., & Bonde, L. O. (Ed.). (2000). *Music in Paediatric Hospitals: Nordic Perspectives*. CREMAH.

Johns, U. (2017). Når musikk skaper nye bevegelsesmuligheter for traumatiserte barn [When music creates new movement possibilities for traumatized children]. In K. Stensæth, G. Trondalen, & Ø. Varkøy (Eds.), *Musikk, handlinger, muligheter: Festskrift til Even Ruud [Even Ruud, Music Therapy in Child Welfare Memorial Volume]* (pp. 107–123). Centre for Music and Health, CREAMAH.

Johnson, K., & Heiderscheit, A. (2018). A survey of music therapy methods on adolescent inpatient mental health units. *Journal of Music Therapy, 55*(4), 463–488. https://doi.org/10.1093/jmt/thy015

Jones, G. (2002). *Killing infants: Angel makers in Europe from the 19th to 20th centuries.* Oxford University Press.

Jones, P., Cedar, L., Coleman, A., Haythorne, D., Mercieca, D., & Ramsden, E. (2021). *Child agency and voice in therapy: New ways of working in the arts therapies.* Routledge.

Jordan, A.-K., Pfeifer, E., Stegemann, T., & Lutz Hochreutener, S. (Eds.). (2018). *Musiktherapie in pädagogischen Settings: Impulse aus Praxis.* Theorie und Forschung.

Kaku, S. M., Sibeoni, J., Basheer, S., et al. (2022). Global child and adolescent mental health perspectives: Bringing change locally, while thinking globally. *Child and Adolescent Psychiatry and Mental Health, 16*(82). https://doi.org/10.1186/s13034-022-00512-8

Kenny, C. (2006). *Music and life in the field of play.* Barcelona Publishers.

Kern, P., & Tague, D. (2017). Music therapy practice status and trends worldwide: An international survey study. *Music Therapy Perspectives, 35*(1), 255–286. https://doi.org/10.1093/jmt/thx011

Kilday, A. M., & Nash, D. (2023). 'Angels of the House' or 'Angel-Makers'? Problematizing murderous mothers in the nineteenth century. *Beyond deviant damsels: Re-evaluating female criminality in the nineteenth century* (Oxford, 2023; online edn, Oxford Academic, March 23, 2023). Retrieved October 1, 2024, from https://doi.org/10.1093/oso/9780198830733.003.0004, .

Kilkelly, U., & Liefaard, T. (2019). International human rights of children. In *International human rights* (pp. 138–154). Springer.

Kim, J., & Stegemann, T. (2016). Music listening for children and adolescents in health care contexts: A systematic review. *The Arts in Psychotherapy, 51*, 72–85. https://s443-doiorg.libdatabase.newpaltz.edu/10.1016/j.aip.2016.08.007

Klyve, G. P. (2019). Whose knowledge? Epistemic injustice and challenges in hearing children's voices. *Voices: A World Forum for Music Therapy, 19*(3).

Klyve, G. P., & Rolvsjord, R. (2023). Moments of fun: Narratives of children's experiences of music therapy in mental health care. *Nordic Journal of Music Therapy, 32*(2), 100–120. https://doi.org/10.1080/08098131.2022.2055114

Klyve, G. P., Rolvsjord, R., & Elgen, I. B. (2023). Polyphonic perspectives: A focus group study of interprofessional staff's perceptions of music therapy at an inpatient unit for children in mental health care. *International Journal of Qualitative Studies on Health and Well-Being, 18*(1), 2197750. https://doi.org/10.1080/17482631.2023.2197750

Knijn, T., & van Nijnatten, C. (2011). Child welfare in The Netherlands: Between privacy and protection. In N. Gilbert, N. Parton, & M. Skivenes (Eds.), *Child protection systems: International trends and orientations* (Online ed.). Oxford Academic. https://doi.org/10.1093/acprof:oso/9780199793358.003.0011

Knoerl, R., Mazzola, E., Woods, H., Buchbinder, E., Frazier, L., laCasce, A., Luskin, M. R., Phillips, C. S., Thornton, K., Berry, D. L., & Ligibel, J. (2023). Exploring influencing factors of anxiety improvement following mindfulness=based music therapy in young adults with cancer. *Journal of Music Therapy, 60*(2), 131–148. https://doi.org/10.1093/jmt/thac017

Knott, D., Biard, M., Nelson, K. E., Epstein, S., Robb, S. L., & Ghetti, C. M. (2020). A survey of music therapists working in pediatric medical settings in the United States. *Journal of Music Therapy, 57*(1), 34–65. https://doi.org/10.1093/jmt/thz019

Koelsch, S. (2015). Music-evoked emotions: Principles, brain correlates, and implications for therapy. *Annals of the New York Academy of Sciences, 1337*, 193–201. https://doi.org/10.1111/nyas.12684

Konieczna-Nowak, L. (2023). Can you hear me now? The potential of trauma-informed and resilience-oriented music therapy in the context of foster care. Open Journal Systems, 7, 153–165. https://doi.org/10.17951/PE/2023.7.153-165

van der Kolk, B. (2014). *The body keeps the score: Brain, mind, and body in the healing of trauma*. Viking.

Krappmann, L. (2010). The weight of the child's view (Article 12 of the Convention on the Rights of the Child). *International Journal of Children's Rights, 18*(4), 501–513.

Krüger, V. (2016). Musikk som ressurs for ungdommers livslange læringsbehov—Et tverrfaglig eksempel fra skolen og barnevernets praksis [Music as a resource for adolescents' life-long learning processes: An interdisciplinary case example from school and child welfare]. In L. Stensæth, V. Krüger, & S. Fuglestad (Eds.), *I transitt mellom til og fra: Tekster om musikk og deltakelse i barnevern [In transit—Between toward and from: Texts about music and participation in a child welfare setting]*. Norwegian Academy of Music.

Krüger, V. (2019). Music as a structuring resource in identity formation processes by adolescents engaging in music therapy—A case story from a Norwegian child welfare setting. In K. McFerran, P. Derrington, & S. Saarikallio (Eds.), *Handbook of music, adolescents, and wellbeing*. Oxford University Press.

Krüger, V. (2020). *Music therapy in child welfare: Bridging provision, protection, and participation*. Barcelona Publishers.

Krüger, V., & Diaz, E. (2023). The potential to meet the needs of refugees and other migrants through music therapy. *The Lancet Regional Health, 29, Article 100637*. https://doi.org/10.1016/j.lancha.2023.100637

Krüger, V., & Stige, B. (2014). Between rights and realities—Music as a structuring resource in the context of child welfare aftercare. A qualitative study. *Nordic Journal of Music Therapy, 24*(2), 1–24.

Krüger, V., & Stige, B. (2015). Between rights and realities–music as a structuring resource in child welfare everyday life: A qualitative study. *Nordic Journal of Music Therapy, 24*(2), 99–122.

Krüger, V., & Tuastad, L. (2025). The Lil Peep paradox—The role of professional discretion when dealing with complex idioms from popular culture. *iNordic Journal of Music Therapy*, 1–16. https://doi.org/10.1080/08098131.2025.2465758

Krüger, V., Nordanger, D. Ø., & Stige. (2018). Music therapy: Building bridges between a participatory approach and trauma-informed care in a child welfare setting. *Voices: A World Forum for Music Therapy, 18*(4) https://voices.no/index.php/voices/article/view/2593

Krüger, V., Risnes, T., Nilsen, C. S., & Høiseth, T. (2019). Musikkterapi og skoledeltakelse for ungdommer med barnevernsbakgrunn—en casestudie [Music therapy and school participation for youth with a child welfare background—A case study]. *Norges Barnevern, 96*(1–2), 40–55.

Krüger, V., Crooke, A., Solberg, D., & Sæle, E. (2023). Exploring the potential for music therapy to support 21st century education goals: Interviews with six Norwegian teachers. *Voices: A World Forum for Music Therapy, 23*(1). https://doi.org/10.15845/voices.v23i1.3642

Krüger, V., Lexander, H., Fyhn, T. & Klette-Bøhler, K. (2024). Musisk medborgerskap –musikkverksted som tilnærming i forebyggende arbeid for unge, en kvalitativ analyse av kommunalt ansattes erfaringer. *Fontene Forskning*. [Musical citizenship—music workshop as an approach in preventive work for young people, a qualitative analysis of municipal employees' experiences]. (Fontene Research).

Langford, M., Skivenes, M., Søvig, K. H., & Loven Kirkebø, T. (2019). Introduction: Implementing child rights. In M. Langford, M. Skivenes, & K. H. Søvig (Eds.), *Children's rights in Norway: An implementation paradox?* (pp. 15–41). Universitetsforlaget.

Lansdown, G. (2011). *Every child's right to be heard: A resource guide on the UN Committee on the Rights of the Child General Comment No.12*. Save the Children/UNICEF.

Lave, J., & Wenger, E. (1991). *Situated learning: Legitimate peripheral participation*. Cambridge University Press.

Lefevre, M. (2004). Finding the key: Containing and processing traumatic sexual abuse. *The Arts in Psychotherapy, 31*(3), 137–152. https://doi.org/10.1016/j.aip.2004.05.001

Lehmann, S., Havik, O., Havik, T., & Heiervang, E. (2013). Mental disorders in foster children: A study of prevalence, comorbidity, and risk factors. *Child and*

Adolescent Psychiatry and Mental Health, 7(39). https://doi.org/10.1186/1753-2000-7-39

Lipsky, M. (2010). *Street-level bureaucracy. Dilemmas of the individual in public services* (30th Anniversary Expanded ed.). Russel Sage Foundation.

Loewy, J. (2015). Medical music therapy for children. In B. L. Wheeler (Ed.), *Music therapy handbook* (pp. 425–440). The Guilford Press.

Loewy, J., Steward, K., Dassler, A.-M., Telsy, A., & Homel, P. (2013). The effects of music therapy on vital signs, feeding, and sleep in premature infants. *Pediatrics, 131*(5), 902–908. https://doi.org/10.1542/peds.2012-1367

Lundy, L. (2007). 'Voice' is not enough: Conceptualising Article 12 of the United Nations Convention on the Rights of the Child. *British Educational Research Journal, 33*(6), 927–942.

Lundy, L., McEvoy, L., & Byrne, B. (2011). Working with young children as co-researchers: An approach informed by the United Nations Convention on the Rights of the Child. *Early Education and Development, 22*(5), 714–736.

Lutz Hochreutener, S. (2018). Musiktherapie im schulischen Kontext. Fakten—Herausforderungen—Chancen. In A. Jordan, E. Pfeifer, T. Stegemann, & S. L. Hochreutener (Eds.), *Musiktherapie in pädagogischen Setting. Impulse aus Praxis, Theorie und Forschung* (pp. 15–30).

MacDonald, R., Kreutz, G., & Mitchell, L. (Eds.). (2013). *Music, health, and wellbeing.* Oxford University Press.

Magee, W. L., Ghetti, C. M., & Moyer, A. (2015). Feasibility of the music therapy assessment tool for awareness in disorders of consciousness (MATADOC) for use with pediatric populations. *Frontiers in Psychology, 6*, 698. https://doi.org/10.3389/fpsyg.2015.00698

Mahoney, E. R. (2015). *Multicultural music therapy: An exploration* [Position paper]. *Voices: A World Forum for Music Therapy, 15*(2). https://doi.org/10.15845/voices.v15i2.832

Mallett, R., & Runswick-Cole, K. (2014). *Approaching disability: Critical issues and perspectives* (1st ed.). Routledge.

Malloch, S., & Trevarthen, C. (Eds.). (2009). *Communicative musicality: Exploring the basis of human companionship* (pp. 357–376). Oxford University Press.

Malone, K., Tesar, M., & Arndt, S. (2020). *Theorising posthuman childhood studies.* Springer.

Mandal, A. B., & Bergset, L. J. (2016). Musikkterapi for å skape samanheng i fosterbarn sine nettverk. [Music therapy to create a connection between the networks of a child in foster care.] In K. Stens.th, V. Krüger, & S. Fuglestad (Eds.), *I transitt—mellom til og fra: Om musikk og deltagelse i barnevern* (pp. 143–156). Anthology published by the Center for Research in Music and Health. Oslo, Norway: Norwegian Academy of Music.

March of Dimes. (2016). *Peristats.* Retrieved from http://www.marchofdimes.org/peristats/whatsnew.aspx?id=42

Marx, K. (1867/1990). *Capital: A critique of political economy* (B. Fowkes, Trans., Vol. 1). Penguin Books. (Original work published 1867).

Massullo, C., De Rossi, E., Carbone, G. A., Imperatori, C., Ardito, R. B., Adenzato, M., & Farina, B. (2023). Child maltreatment, abuse, and neglect: An umbrella review of their prevalence and definitions. *Clinical Neuropsychiatry, 20*(2), 72–99. https://doi.org/10.36131/cnfioritieditore20230201

Masten, A. S., & Tellegen, A. (2012). Resilience in developmental psychopathology: Contributions of the project competence longitudinal study. *Development and Psychopathology, 24*(2), 345–361. https://doi.org/10.1017/S095457941200003X

Mastroianni, A. C., Faden, R., & Federman, D. (Eds.). (1994). *Institute of medicine (US) committee on ethical and legal issues relating to the inclusion of women in clinical studies.* National Academies Press. https://www.ncbi.nlm.nih.gov/books/NBK236544/

Mata Ferro, M., Falcó-Pegueroles, A., Fernández-Lorenzo, R., Saz-Roy, M. A., Rodríguez-Forner, O., Estrada Jurado, C. M., Bonet Julià, N., Geli Benito, C., Hernádez Hernáde, R., & Bosch Alcaraz, A. (2023). The effect of a live music therapy intervention on critically ill paediatric patients in the intensive care unit: A quasi-experimental pretest-posttest study. *Australian Critical Care, 36*(6), 967–973. https://doi.org/10.1016/j.aucc.2023.01.006

McFerran, K. S. (2010). *Adolescents, music, and music therapy: Methods and techniques for clinicians, educators, and students.* Jessica Kingsley Publishers.

McFerran, K. S. (2020). Adolescents and music therapy: Contextualized recommendations for research and practice. *Music Therapy Perspectives, 38*(1), 80–88. https://doi.org/10.1093/mtp/miz014

McFerran, K. S., & Crooke, A. (2014). Enabling tailored music programs in elementary schools: An Australian exemplar. *Journal of Education and Training Studies, 2*(4). https://doi.org/10.11114/jets.v2i4.536

McFerran, K. S., & Saarikallio, S. (2014). Depending on music to feel better: Being conscious of responsibility when appropriating the power of music. *The Arts in Psychotherapy, 41*, 89–97. https://doi.org/10.1016/j.aip.2014.01.007

McFerran, K. S., & Shoemark, H. (2013). How musical engagement promotes well-being in education contexts: The case of a young man with profound and multiple disabilities. *International Journal of Qualitative Studies on Health and Well-Being, 8*, 20570. https://doi.org/10.3402/qhw.v8i0.2057

McFerran, K., & Stephenson, J. (2010). Facing the challenge: A music therapy investigation in the evidence-based framework. In V. Karkou (Ed.), *Arts therapies in schools: Research and practice* (pp. 259–270). Jessica Kingsley Publishers.

McFerran, K. S., & Teggelove, T. (2011). Music therapy with young people in schools: After the Black Saturday fires. *Voices: A World Forum for Music Therapy, 11*(1).

McFerran, K., Roberts, M., & O'Grady, L. (2010). Music therapy with bereaved teenagers: A mixed methods perspective. *Death Studies, 34*(6), 541–565. https://doi.org/10.1080/07481181003765428

McFerran, K. S., Hense, C., Koike, A., & Rickwood, D. (2018). Intentional music use to reduce psychological distress in adolescents accessing primary mental health care. *Clinical Child Psychology and Psychiatry, 23*(4), 567–581. https://doi.org/10.1177/1359104518767231

McIntyre, J. (2009). Interactive family music therapy: Untangling the system. *The Australian and New Zealand Journal of Family Therapy, 30*(4), 260–268. https://doi.org/10.1375/anft.30.4.260

McLaughlin, J., Coleman-Fountain, E., & Clavering, E. (2016). *Disabled childhoods: Monitoring differences and emerging identities* (1st ed.). Routledge. https://doi.org/10.4324/9781315795898

Medina, J. (2018). Misrecognition and epistemic injustice. *Feminist Philosophy Quarterly, 4*(4). https://doi.org/10.5206/fpq/2018.4.6233

Merriam-Webster. (n.d.). Autonomy. In Merriam-Webster.com dictionary. Retrieved August 13, 2024, from https://www.merriam-webster.com/dictionary/autonomy

Metell, M. (2014). Disabling musicking: Reflections on a disability studies perspective in music therapy. *Voices: A World Forum for Music Therapy, 14*(3). https://doi.org/10.15845/voices.v14i3.786

Metell, M. (2019). How we talk when we talk about disabled children and their families: An invitation to queer the discourse. *Voices: A World Forum for Music Therapy, 19*(3). https://doi.org/10.15845/voices.v19i3.2652

Metell, M. (2023). *Disabled children's access to music.* Music's Transform.

Metell, M., & Leza, J. (2023). Exploring queer theories as a framework for anti-oppressive music therapy practice with neurodivergent children and youth. In C. A. Lee (Ed.), *The Oxford handbook of queer and trans music therapy* (pp. 370–385). Oxford University Press. https://doi.org/10.1093/oxfordhb/9780192898364.013.21

Miell, D. E., MacDonald, R. A. R., & Hargreaves, D. J. (2005). *Musical communication.* Oxford University Press.

Miles, S. H. (2004). *The Hippocratic oath and the ethics of medicine.* Oxford University Press.

Ministèrio da Educação. (2024). *Orientações para Creche* [Direção-Geral da Educação]. https://www.dge.mec.pt/sites/default/files/opc_marco2024.pdf

Ministry of Education of the People's Republic of China. (2012). *Guideline for learning and development of children aged 3–6.* Beijing, China: Ministry of Education. https://www.unicef.cn/sites/unicef.org.china/files/2018-10/2012-national-early-learning-development-guidelines.pdf),

Mitchell, E. (2019). Community music therapy and participatory performance: Case study of a coffee house. *Voices: A World Forum for Music Therapy, 19*(1). https://doi.org/10.15845/voices.v19i1.2701

Mitchell, E. (2021). Performing identities and performing relationships: Community music therapy and adolescent mental health. *Music Therapy Perspectives, 39*(2), 195–203. https://doi.org/10.1093/mtp/miab004

Mitchell, E. (2023). Music's relational imperative: Wellbeing, music-making, and the interconnections between music therapy and music education. In K. S. Hendricks (Ed.), *The Oxford handbook of care in music education* (pp. 361–372). Oxford University Press. https://doi.org/10.1093/oxfordhb/9780197611654.013.33

Mojtabai, R., & Olfson, M. (2024). Trends in mental disorders in children and adolescents receiving treatment in the state mental health system. *Journal of the American Academy of Child & Adolescent Psychiatry*, PMID 39214290. https://doi.org/10.1016/j.jaac.2024.08.008

Molander, A. (2016). *Discretion in the welfare state: Social rights and professional judgment.* Routledge.

Mössler, K., Halstead, J., Metell, M., Gottschewski, K., & Schmid, W. (2022). "The room is a mess": Exploring the co-creation of space for attunement dynamics between an autistic child and a non-autistic music therapist. *Nordic Journal of Music Therapy*, 1–21. https://doi.org/10.1080/08098131.2022.2145346

Munro, E. (2011). *Munro review of child protection, final report: A child-centred system.* Department for Education.

Murris, K. (2016). *The posthuman child: Educational transformation through philosophy with picturebooks.* Routledge. https://doi.org/10.4324/9781315714405

National Commission for the Protection of Human Subjects of Biomedical and Behavioral Research. (1979). *The Belmont report: Ethical principles and guidelines for the protection of human subjects of research.* U.S. Department of Health, Education, and Welfare. https://www.hhs.gov/ohrp/regulations-and-policy/belmont-report/index.html

Nhan Nguyen, T., Nilsson, S., Hellström, A.-L., & Bengtson, A. (2010). Music therapy to reduce pain and anxiety in children with cancer undergoing lumbar puncture: A randomized clinical trial. *Journal of Pediatric Oncology Nursing, 27*(3), 146–155.

Nicholson, J. M., Berthelsen, D., Abad, V., Williams, K., & Bradley, J. (2008). Impact of music therapy to promote positive parenting and child development. *Journal of Health Psychology, 13*(2), 226–238. https://doi.org/10.1177/1359105307086705

Nilsson, S., Kokinsky, E., Nilsson, U., Sidenvall, B., & Enskär, K. (2009). School-aged children's experience of postoperative music medicine on pain, distress and anxiety. *Pediatric Anesthesia, 19*, 1184–1190.

Nöcker-Ribaupierre, M., & Wölfl, A. (2010). Music to counter violence: A preventative approach for working with adolescents in schools. *Nordic Journal of Music Therapy, 19*(2), 151–161. https://doi.org/10.1080/08098131.2010.489997

Noguchi, L. K. (2006). The effect of music versus nonmusic on behavioral signs of distress and self-report of pain in pediatric injection patients. *Journal of Music Therapy, 43*, 16–38.

Nordoff, P., & Robbins, C. (1971). *Music therapy in special education* (p. 253). John Day Company.

Office of the High Commissioner United Nations Human Rights. (1989). *Convention of the rights of the child*. https://www.ohchr.org/en/instruments-mechanisms/instruments/convention-rights-child

Oldfield, A. (2017). The first 'themed' British journal of music therapy: An introduction to music therapy with families. *British Journal of Music Therapy, 31*(1), 5–11. https://doi.org/10.1177/1359457517697808

Oosthuizen, H. B. (2018). Working with and within chaos: The development of a music therapy program for young sex offenders in South Africa. *Voices: A World Forum for Music Therapy, 18*(4). https://doi.org/10.15845/voices.v18i4.2588

Oranga Tamariki Act. 1989/2019, No 24 (as amended in 2019). Retrieved from https://www.legislation.govt.nz/act/public/1989/0024/latest/DLM147088.html

Oselame, M. do N. (2023). *"No não sentir não há sentido": A musicoterapia como uma prática de cuidado em saúde no sistema socioeducativo* (Doctoral thesis). Fundação Oswaldo Cruz—Escola Nacional de Saúde Pública Sergio Arouca.

Özgürbüz, N., Bahar, A., Tuna, A., & Çopur, E. (2024). The effect of lullaby played to preterm infants in neonatal intensive care units on physiological parameters and pain. *Journal of Pediatric Nursing, 79*, 133–140. https://doi.org/10.1016/j.pedn.2024.08.019

Parsons, J. (2022). Whose "power of music"? Questioning and problematizing aspects of language and power in music therapy practice within mainstream primary schools in the UK. *Voices: A World Forum for Music Therapy, 22*(3). https://doi.org/10.15845/voices.v22i3.3406

Pasiali, V. (2017). Families and children at risk. In S. L. Jacobsen & G. Thompson (Eds.), *Music therapy with families: Therapeutic approaches and theoretical perspectives*. Jessica Kingsley.

Pavlicevic, M. (2003). *Groups in music: Strategies from music therapy*. Jessica Kingsley Publishers.

PediStat. (2024, July 1). *What is the age range for pediatrics?* https://www.pedistat.com/blog/what-the-age-range-for-pediatrics

Pèrez-Eizaguirre, M., Dorado, A., Rodríguez-Brioso, M., & Privado, J. (2022). Efficacy of music therapy in the treatment of anxiety among children at social risk and those have committed child to parent violence. *Psychology of Music, 50*(1), 328–342.

Perryman, K., Blisard, P., & Moss, R. (2019). Using creative arts in trauma therapy: The neuroscience of healing. *Journal of Mental Health Counseling, 41*(1), 80–94. https://doi.org/10.17744/mehc.41.1.07

Pethybridge, E., & Robertson, J. (2010). Educational music therapy: Theoretical foundations explored in time-limited group work projects with children. In V. Karkou (Ed.), *Arts therapies in schools: Research and practice* (pp. 129–144). Jessica Kingsley Publishers.

Pieper, L., & Thomson, C. J. H. (2013). Justice in human research ethics. A conceptual and practice guide. *Monash Bioethics Review, 31*(1), 91–116.

Polanyi, M. (1967). *The tacit dimension* (Vol. A540, pp. xi, 108). Doubleday.

Porter, S., McConnell, T., McLaughlin, K., Lynn, F., Cardwell, C., Braiden, H. J., Boylan, J., & Holmes, V. (2017). Music therapy for children and adolescents with behavioural and emotional problems: A randomised controlled trial. *The Journal of Child Psychology and Psychiatry, 58*(5), 586–594.

Powell, M. A., & Smith, A. S. (2009). Children's participation rights in research. *Childhood, 16*(1), 124–142. https://doi.org/10.1177/0907566208101694

Pratt, B., Wild, V., Barasa, E., Kamuya, D., Gilson, L., Hendl, T., & Molyneux, S. (2020). Justice: A key consideration in health policy and systems research ethics. *BMJ Global Health, 5*, e001942. https://doi.org/10.1136/bmjgh-2019-001942

Priestley, M. (1994). *Essays on analytical music therapy*. Barcelona Publishers.

Preyde, M., Berends, A., Parekh, S., & Heintzman, J. (2015). Adolescents' evaluation of music therapy in an inpatient psychiatric unit: A quality improvement project. *Music Therapy Perspectives, 35*(1), 58–62. https://doi.org/10.1093/mtp/miv027

Radez, J., Reardon, T., Creswell, C., Lawrence, P. J., Evdoka-Burton, G., & Waite, P. (2021). Why do children and adolescents (not) seek and access professional help for their mental health problems? A systematic review of quantitative and qualitative studies. *European Child & Adolescent Psychiatry, 30*(2), 183–211. https://doi.org/10.1007/s00787-019-01469-4

Regulation (EU) 2016/679. (2016, April 27). Regulation (EU) 2016/679 of the European Parliament and of the Council of 27 April 2016 on the protection of natural persons with regard to the processing of personal data and on the free movement of such data, and repealing Directive 95/46/EC (General Data Protection Regulation). *Official Journal of the European Union, L 119*, 1–88. https://eur-lex.europa.eu/eli/reg/2016/679/ojWikipedia+2Academia Stack Exchange+2

Rickson, D. (2012). Music therapy school consultation: A unique practice. *Nordic Journal of Music Therapy, 21*(3), 268–285. https://doi.org/10.1080/08098131.2012.654474

Rickson, D., & McFerran, K. (2014). *Creating music cultures in the schools: A perspective from community music therapy*. Barcelona Publishers.

Roaldsnes, M. H. (2017). *Musikk i helsefremmande arbeid med einslege mindreårige flyktningar. Ein kvalitativ studie av ei musikkgruppe for ungdom med bakgrunn som einslege flyktningbarn* [Music in health promoting work with unaccompanied minor refugees. A qualitative study of a music group for adolescents with a background as unaccompanied minor refugees] (Doctoral dissertation). Norwegian Academy of Music. https://brage.bibsys.no/xmlui/bitstream/handle/11250/2469525/RoaldsneAvhandling_nett.pdf

Robb, S. L., & Carpenter, J. S. (2009). A review of music-based intervention reporting in pediatrics. *Journal of Health Psychology, 14*(4), 490–501. https://doi.org/10.1177/1359105309103568

Rolvsjord, R. (2010). *Resource-oriented music therapy in mental health care*. Barcelona Publishers.

Rosado, A. (2019). Adolescents' experiences of music therapy on an inpatient crisis stabilization unit. *Music Therapy Perspectives, 37*(2), 133–140. https://doi.org/10.1093/mtp/miz004

Rossetti, A. (2020). Environmental Music Therapy (EMT): Music's contribution to changing hospital atmospheres and perceptions of environments. *Music and Medicine, 12*(2), 130–141. https://s443-doiorg.libdatabase.newpaltz.edu/10.47513/mmd.v12i2.742

Ross, W. D., & Brown, L. (2009). *The Nicomachean ethics*. Oxford University Press.

Roth, L. H., Meisel, A., & Lidz, C. W. (1977). Test of competency to consent to treatment. *American Journal of Psychiatry, 124*, 279–284.

Ruggiero, R. (2022). Article 3: The Best Interest of the Child, In Vaghri, Z. (2022). Monitoring state compliance with the UN Convention on the rights of the child. *Children's Well-Being: Indicators and Research, 25*. https://doi.org/10.1007/978-3-030-84647-3_3

Ruud, E. (1998). *Music therapy, improvisation, communication, and culture*. Barcelona Publishers.

Ruud, E. (2010). *Music therapy: A perspective from the humanities*. Barcelona Publishers.

Saarikallio, S. (2019). Music as a resource for agency and empowerment in identity construction. In K. McFerran, P. Derrington, & S. Saarikallio (Eds.), *Handbook of music, adolescents, and well-being* (pp. 89–99). Oxford University Press.

Salari, N., Heidarian, P., Hassanabadi, M., et al. (2024). Global prevalence of social anxiety disorder in children, adolescents and youth: A systematic review and meta-analysis. *Journal of Prevention*. https://doi.org/10.1007/s10935-024-00789-9

Santos, A. D. (2018). Empathy and aggression in group music therapy with teenagers: A descriptive phenomenological study. *Music Therapy Perspectives*. Advance online publication. https://doi.org/10.1093/mtp/miy024.

dos Santos, A. (2019). Empathy and aggression in group music therapy with teenagers: A descriptive phenomenological study. *Music Therapy Perspectives, 37*(1), 14–27. https://doi.org/10.1093/mtp/miy024

dos Santos, A. (2024). Nurturing our reflexivity. *Nordic Journal of Music Therapy, 33*(1), 1–3. https://doi.org/10.1080/08098131.2023.2282814

Save the children. (2021). *Fritid for alle—uten fordommer. Fortellinger om fritid fra barn og ungdom med funksjonsnedsettelse [Leisure time for everyone –without prejudices. Narratives on leisure time from children and youth with disability].*

Schön, D. A. (1983). *The reflective practitioner: How professionals think in action.* Basic Books.

Schrader, E. M., & Wendland, J. M. (2012). Music therapy programming at an aftercare center in Cambodia for survivors of child sexual exploitation and rape and their caregivers. *Social Work & Christianity, 39*(4), 390–406.

Scrine, E. (2019). Reframing intervention and inclusion: The importance of exploring gender and sexuality in music therapy with all young people. In *Handbook of music, adolescents, and wellbeing* (pp. 151–161). Oxford University Press.

Scrine, E. (2021). The limits of resilience and the need for resistance: Articulating the role of music therapy with young people within a shifting trauma paradigm. *Frontiers in Psychology, 12*, 600245. https://doi.org/10.3389/fpsyg.2021.600245

Sen, S. (2017). *Image: No child left invisible.* Harper Collins.

Shaw, C. M. (2022). An autoethnographic journey in developing post-ableist music therapy. *Voices: A World Forum for Music Therapy, 22*(1). https://doi.org/10.15845/voices.v22i1.3314

Shaw, C., & Metell, M. (in press). Music therapy and disability. In I. B. Wheeler, M. Viega, & A. dos Santos (Eds.), *Music therapy handbook.* Guildford Press.

Shelton, L. (2019). *The Bronfenbrenner primer: A guide to develecology.* Routledge.

Shoemark, H. (2013). Full term hospitalized newborns. In J. Bradt (Ed.), *Guidelines for music therapy practice in pediatric care* (pp. 116–151). Barcelona Publishers.

Shoemark, H., Rimmer, J., Bower, J., Tucquet, B., Miller, L., Fisher, M., Ogburn, N., & Dun, B. (2018). A conceptual framework: The musical self as a unique pathway to outcomes in the acute pediatric health setting. *Journal of Music Therapy, 55*(1), 1–26. https://doi.org/10.1093/jmt/thx018

Shuman, J., Kennedy, H., DeWitt, P., Edelblute, A., & Wamboldt, M. Z. (2016). Group music therapy impacts mood states of adolescents in a psychiatric hospital setting. *The Arts in Psychotherapy, 49*, 50–56. https://doi.org/10.1016/j.aip.2016.03.001

Siegel, D. J. (2012). *The developing mind: How relationships and the brain interact to shape who we are* (3rd ed.). Guilford Press.

Simensen, E. (Ed.). (2021). *The older Gulathing law* (1st ed., Chapter 21). Routledge.

Sinclair, R. (2004). Participation in practice: Making it meaningful, effective, and sustainable. *Children & Society, 18*, 106–118.

Siu, A., & Robinson, C. A. (2014). Neonatal abstinence syndrome: essentials for the practitioner. *The Journal of Pediatric Pharmacology and Therapeutics : JPPT: The Official Journal of PPAG, 19*(3), 147–155. https://s443-doiorg.libdatabase.newpaltz.edu/10.5863/1551-6776-19.3.147

Skivenes, M., & Sørsdal, L. M. (2018). The child's best interest principle across child protection jurisdictions. In A. Falch-Eriksen & E. Backe-Hansen (Eds.), *Human rights in child protection* (pp. 59–88). Palgrave Macmillan. https://doi.org/10.1007/978-3-319-94800-3_4

Skogdal, E. (2015). Hvem får være musikkelev?—Kunstdidaktisk eller terapeutisk ståsted [Who gets to be a music student? Art didactic or therapeutic standpoint]. *Nordic Journal of Art & Research, 4*(2).

Small, C. (1998). *Musicking: The meanings of performing and listening*. Wesleyan University Press.

Smith, A., Caine, K., & Hanson-Abromeit, D. (2018). Music therapy for neonatal intensive care. In A. Knight, B. laGasse, & A. Clair (Eds.), *Music therapy: An Introduction to the profession* (pp. 247–264). American Music Therapy Association.

Sokira, J., Allen, J., & Wagner, H. (2023). The resilience framework for trauma-informed music therapy. In L. Beer & J. C. Birnbaum (Eds.), *Trauma-informed music therapy* (pp. 9–18). Routledge.

Spandler, H. (2024). "What matters to you?"—An antidote to "What's wrong" and "What happened". *Mad in America: Science, psychiatry and social justice.*

Stanley, J. M., & Walworth, D. (2010). *Music therapy with premature infants: Research and developmental interventions* (2nd ed.). American Music Therapy Association.

Steele, M., McFerran, K. S., & Crooke, A. H. D. (2019). Reconceptualizing music therapist/teacher consultation: Supporting teachers through a music for well-being professional learning program. *Voices: A World Forum for Music Therapy.*

Stegemann, T., Geretsegger, M., Phan Quoc, E., Riedl, H., & Smetana, M. (2019). Music therapy and other music-based interventions in pediatric health care: An overview. *Medicine, 6*(1), 25. https://doi.org/10.3390/medicines6010025

Steinhardt, T. L., Mortvedt, S., & Trondalen, G. (2021). Music therapy in the hospital-at-home: A practice for children in palliative care. *British Journal of Music Therapy, 35*(2), 53–62. https://doi.org/10.1177/13594575211029109

Stern, D. N. (2010). *Forms of vitality: Exploring dynamic experience in psychology, the arts, psychotherapy, and development*. Oxford University Press.

Stige, B. (2002). *Culture-centered music therapy*. Barcelona Publishers.

Stige, B., & Aarø, L. E. (2012). *Invitation to community music therapy*. Routledge.

Storsve, V., Westbye, I. A., & Ruud, E. (2010). Hope and recognition: A music project among youth in a Palestinian refugee camp. *Voices: A World Forum for. Music Therapy, 10*(1). https://doi.org/10.15845/voices.v10i1.158

Strehlow, G. (2009). The use of music therapy in treating sexually abused children. *Nordic Journal of Music Therapy, 18*(2), 167–183. https://doi.org/10.1080/08098130903062397

Stuart, K. (2018). Musical ripples and reflections: The story of Charlie, his music, and his new foster family. *Voices: A World Forum for Music Therapy, 18*(4). https://doi.org/10.15845/voices.v18i4.2886

Sturman, E. D. (2005). The capacity to consent to treatment and research: A review of standardized assessment tools. *Clinical Psychology Review, 25*(7), 954–974.

Substance Abuse and Mental Health Services Administration [SAMHSA]. (2014). *SAMHSA's concept of trauma and guidance for a trauma-informed approach*. HHS Publication No. (SMA) 14–4884. Author.

Sullivan, L. N. (2003). Meet them in the lab: Using hip-hop music therapy groups with adolescents in residential settings. In N. E. Sullivan, E. S. Mesbur, N. C. Lang, D. Goodman, & L. Mitchell (Eds.), *Social work with groups: Social justice through personal, community, and societal change* (pp. 103–116). The Haworth Press, Inc.

Sutton, J. (2002). Trauma in context. In J. Sutton (Ed.), *Music, music therapy, and trauma: International perspectives* (pp. 21–41). Jessica Kingsley Publishers.

Suzuki, D. C., Monge, A., Silva, B. S., Viana, J. A., Suzuki, P. R., Annunciato Neto, R., & Vitalle, M. S. (2023). *Adolescent victims of sexual abuse and music therapy: A systematic review*. Research, Society and Development.

Tabinowski, K. (2013). *A survey of current music therapy practices in pediatric hospitals and units* [Unpublished master's thesis]. Florida State University.

Tan, L., Kocsis, A., & Burry, J. (2023). Advancing Donald Schön's reflective practitioner: Where to next? *Design Issues, 39*(3), 3–18. https://doi.org/10.1162/desi_a_00722

Teachout, D. J. (2005). The impact of music education on a child's growth and development. Sounds of learning. *International Foundation for Music Research, 46*(4), 568–587.

Teggelove, K., Thompson, G., & Tamplin, J. (2019). Supporting positive parenting practices within a community-based music therapy group program: Pilot study findings. *Journal of Community Psychology, 47*(4), 712–726. https://doi.org/10.1002/jcop.22148

Thomson, A., Hariss, E., Peters-Corbett, A., Koppel, K., & Creswell, C. (2023). Barriers and facilitators of community-based implementation of evidence-based interventions in the UK, for children and young people's mental health promotion, prevention and treatment: Rapid scoping review. *BJPsych Open, 9*, e132, 1–8. https://doi.org/10.1192/bjo.2023.531

Toader, C., Tataru, C. P., Florian, I. A., Covache-Busuioc, R. A., Bratu, B. G., Glavan, L. A., Bordeianu, A., Dumitrascu, D. I., & Ciurea, A. V. (2023). Cognitive crescendo: How music shapes the brain's structure and function. *Brain Sciences, 13*(10), 1390. https://doi.org/10.3390/brainsci13101390

Trehub, S. E., Becker, J., & Morley, I. (2015). Cross-cultural perspectives on music and musicality. *Philosophical Transactions of the Royal Society of London. Series B, Biological Sciences, 370*(1664), 20140096. https://doi.org/10.1098/rstb.2014.0096

Trondalen, G. (2016). *Relational music therapy: An intersubjective perspective.* Barcelona Publishers.

Tuomi, K., Thompson, G., Gottfried, T., & Ala-Ruona, E. (2021). Theoretical perspectives and therapeutic approaches in music therapy with families. *Voices: A World Forum for Music Therapy, 21*(2). https://doi.org/10.15845/voices.v21i2.2952

Tushnet, M. (1992). The critique of rights. *Southern Methodist University Law Review, 47*, 23–34.

Uggla, L., Bonde, L. O., Svahn, B. M., et al. (2016). Music therapy can lower the heart rates of severely sick children. *Acta Paediatrica, 105*(11), 1225–1230. https://doi.org/10.1111/apa.13452

Uggla, L., Bonde, L.-O., Hammar, U., Wrangsjo, B., & Gustafsson, B. (2018). Music therapy supported the health-related quality of life for children undergoing haematopoietic stem cell transplants. *Acta Paediatrica, 107*, 1986–1994. https://doi.org/10.1111/apa.14515

Uggla, L., Mårtenson Blom, K., Bonde, L. O., et al. (2019). An explorative study of qualities in interactive processes with children and their parents in music therapy during and after pediatric hematopoietic stem cell transplantation. *Medicine, 6*(1), 28. https://doi.org/10.3390/medicines6010028

Uhlig, S., Jansen, E., & Scherder, E. (2018). "Being a bully isn't very cool…": Rap & sing music therapy for enhanced emotional self-regulation in an adolescent school setting - a randomized controlled trial. *Psychology of Music, 46*(4), 568–587. https://doi.org/10.1177/0305735617719154

Ullsten, A., Eriksson, M., Klässbo, M., & Volgsten, U. (2017a). Live music therapy with lullaby singing as affective support during painful procedures: A case study with microanalysis. *Nordic Journal of Music Therapy, 26*(2), 142–166. https://doi.org/10.1080/08098131.2015.1131187

Ullsten, A., Hugoson, P., Forsberg, M., Forzelius, L., Klässbo, M., Olsson, E., et al. (2017b). Efficacy of live lullaby singing during procedural pain in preterm and term neonates. *Music and Medicine: An Interdisciplinary Journal, 9*(2), 73–85.

UN Committee on the Rights of Persons with Disabilities. (2016). *General Comment No. 4 (2016) on the Right to Inclusive Education.* Retrieved from https://www.ohchr.org/en/treaty-bodies/crpd

UN Committee on the Rights of the Child (UNCRC). (2013). *General comment No. 14 on the right of the child to have his or her best interests taken as a primary consideration (art. 3, para. 1).* CRC/C/GC/14. Retrieved from https://www2.ohchr.org/english/bodies/crc/docs/gc/crc_c_gc_14_eng.pdf

UNCHR. (2008). *Guidelines on determining the best interests of the child*. https://www.unhcr.org

UNESCO & United Nations Children's Fund. (2024). *Global report on early childhood care and education: The right to a strong foundation*. https://doi.org/10.54675/FWQA2113.

Unger, R. M. (1986). *The critical legal studies movement*. Harvard University Press.

UNICEF. (2013). *General Comment No. 14 on the Right of the Child to have his or her best interests taken as a primary consideration (Art. 3, para. 1)*. Retrieved from https://www.refworld.org/legal/general/crc/2013/en/95780

UNICEF & World Health Organization. (n.d.). *Nurturing care for early childhood development: A framework for helping children survive and thrive to transform health and human potential*. Retrieved from https://www.unicef.org/reports/nurturing-care-early-childhood-development

UNICEF Office of Research – Innocenti. (n.d.-a). *Towards a child-centred digital equity framework*. UNICEF. https://www.unicef.org/innocenti/media/731/file/UNICEF-Global-Insight-Towards-a-child-centred-digital-equity-framework.pdf

UNICEF Office of Research – Innocenti. (n.d.-b). *Towards a child-centred digital equity framework*. UNICEF. Retrieved from https://www.unicef.org/innocenti/reports/towards-child-centred-digital-equality-framework

United Nations. (1989). *Convention on the rights of the child*. https://www.ohchr.org/en/instruments-mechanisms/instruments/convention-rights-child

United Nations. (2009). *Guidelines for the alternative care of children*. Retrieved from https://digitallibrary.un.org/record/673583?ln=en&v=pdf

United Nations General Assembly. (1959). *Declaration of the Rights of the Child*. Retrieved from https://digitallibrary.un.org/record/195831?ln=en&v=pdf

United Nations General Assembly. (2007). *Convention on the rights of persons with disabilities*. United Nations. Retrieved from https://social.desa.un.org/issues/disability/crpd/convention-on-the-rights of-persons-with-disabilities-crpd

Urban, M., Fairchild, N., Vandenbroeck, M., Lenz Taguchi, H., & Macrine, S. (Eds.). (2022). *Reconceptualising children's rights in infant-toddler care and education: Transnational conversations*. Springer. https://doi.org/10.1007/978-3-031-05218-7

Utdanningsdirektoratet. (2017). *Læreplan*. Utdanningsdirektoratet. https://www.udir.no

Văduva, L. P., & Balla, A. (2019). A study of the efficiency of music therapy, art and play therapy on hospitalized children diagnosed with chronic illnesses. *Studia Universitatis Babes-Bolvai-Musica, 64*(2), 147–160.

Van Rooyen, A., & Dos Santos, A. (2020). Exploring the lived experiences of teenagers in a children's home participating in a choir: A community music therapy perspective. *International Journal of Community Music, 13*(1), Article 00011. https://doi.org/10.1386/ijcm_00011_1

Vatnedalen Vik, A. L., Thiedemann, M., & Brennskag Nettum, L. (2023). Synd med beina, dans med øynene—sangens muligheter li å inkludere alle. In A. H. Balsnes, L. A. Hagen, & S. Haukenes (Eds.), *Sangglede og stemmebruk i barnehagen* (pp. 135–148).

Victorian Government, Department of Health and Human Services. (2018). *Home Stretch Program*. Retrieved from https://www.vic.gov.au/homestretch

Viega, M. (2011). The hero's journey in hip-hop and its applications in music therapy. In S. Hadley & G. Yancy (Eds.), *Therapeutic uses of rap and hip-hop* (p. 22). Routledge. https://doi.org/10.4324/9780203806012

Viega, M. (2016). Exploring the discourse in hip-hop and implications for music therapy practice. *Music Therapy Perspectives, 34*(2), 138–146. https://doi.org/10.1093/mtp/miv035

Vygotsky, L. (1978). *Mind in society: The development of higher psychological processes.* Harvard University Press.

Walker, M. (2002). Autonomy, beneficence, and justice in the wider context. *Ethics and Behavior, 12*, 291–293.

Wang, Y., Li, H.-L., Yang, T., Sung, H.-C., & Huang, H.-M. (2012). The application of music therapy for children and adolescents with mood disorders. *West China Medical Journal, 3*, 423–430. https://doi.org/10.3969/j.issn.1672-1654.2012.04.006

Weber, M. (1978). In G. Roth & C. Wittich (Eds.), *Economy and society: An outline of interpretive sociology.* University of California Press.

Weiss, C., & Bensimon, M. (2019). Group music therapy with uprooted teenagers: The importance of structure. *Nordic Journal of Music Therapy, 29*(1), 20–35. https://doi.org/10.1080/08098131.2019.1695281

West, D. (1998). Radiation experiments on children at the Fernald and Wrentham schools: Lessons for human subject research. *Accountability in Research: Policies & Quality Assurance, 6*(1/2), 103–125.

Wilhelmsen, C., & Fuhr, G. (2018). Reflections on practice: Three examples of relational music therapy practice with adolescents in child welfare services. *Voices: A World Forum for Music Therapy, 18*(4).

Winnicott, D. W. (2005). *Playing and reality* (2nd ed.). Routledge.

Winter, P. (2015). Perspectives on the practice of community music therapy in rural primary schools of Malawi. *Nordic Journal of Music Therapy, 24*(3), 276–287. https://doi.org/10.1080/08098131.2014.964752

Wölfl, A. (2014). *Gewaltprävention mit Musik: Empirische Wirkungsanalyse eines musiktherapeutischen Projektmodells.* Reichert.

World Health Organization. (n.d.). *Mental health.* World Health Organization. https://www.who.int/health-topics/mental-health#tab=tab_1

World Health Organization (WHO). (2011). *Standards and operational guidance for ethics review of health-related research with human participants.* https://www.who.int/publications/i/item/9789241502948

World Health Organization (WHO). (2024, October 10). *Mental health of adolescents.* https://www.who.int/news-room/fact-sheets/detail/adolescent-mental-health

World Medical Association. (2013). *WMA declaration of Helsinki—Ethical principles for medical research involving human subjects.*

World Medical Association. https://www.wma.net/policies-post/wma-declaration-of-helsinki-ethical-principles-for-medical-research-involving-human-subjects/å.

Wyness, M. G. (2012). *Childhood and society: An introduction to the sociology of childhood.* Palgrave Macmillan. https://doi.org/10.1007/978-0-230-24182-4

Ye, P., Huang, Z., Zhou, H., & Tang, Q. (2021). Music-based intervention to reduce aggressive behavior in children and adolescents: A meta-analysis. *Medicine, 100*(4), e23894. https://doi.org/10.1097/MD.0000000000023894

Yinger, O. S., & Gooding, L. F. (2015). A systematic review of music-based intervention for procedural support. *Journal of Music Therapy, 52*(1), 1–77. https://doi.org/10.1093/jmt/thv004

Yinger, O. S., & Lownds, K. (2018). Music therapy in pediatric medicine. In A. Knight, B. laGasse, & A. Clair (Eds.), *Music therapy: An Introduction to the profession* (pp. 265–280). American Music Therapy Association.

Yun, J., & Chong, H. J. (2019). At-risk adolescents' inner resource through resource-oriented song psychotherapy. *Journal of Music and Human Behavior, 16*(2),1–25.https://koreascience.or.kr/article/JAKO201908071719175.page

Zanders, M. L. (2012). The musical and personal biographies of adolescents with foster care experience. In *Collected work: Qualitative inquiries in music therapy. VII* (pp. 71–109). Barcelona Publishers.

Zanders, M. L. (2015). Music therapy practices and processes with foster-care youth: Formulating an approach to clinical work. *Music Therapy Perspectives, 33*(2), 97–107.

Zanders, M. L., Midach, M., Waldmeier, L., & Barros, B. (2018). A reflexive music therapy clinical introspection in working with foster care youth. *Voices: A World Forum for Music Therapy, 18*(4).

Index[1]

[1] Note: Page numbers followed by 'n' refer to notes.

V. Krüger, K. M. Murphy, *Child-Centred Music Therapy*,
https://doi.org/10.1007/978-3-031-85724-9

FSC
www.fsc.org
MIX
Papier | Fördert gute Waldnutzung
FSC® C083411

Kolibri 360 GmbH
Ferdinand-Jühlke-Straße 7
99095 Erfurt, Deutschland
produktsicherheit@kolibri360.de